HIV/AIDS
in the Caribbean
Issues and Options

The World Bank
Washington, D.C.

TABLE OF CONTENTS

BOXES, FIGURES, AND TABLES

BOXES

FIGURES

TABLES

ACKNOWLEDGMENTS

This report was prepared by Patricio V. Marquez, Lead Health Specialist, Human Development Sector Management Unit (LCSHD), Latin America and Caribbean Region, World Bank, with contributions from Victor H. Sierra, Public Health Specialist, Consultant; Jacob Gayle, Senior Technical Advisor, Joint United Nations Program on AIDS (UNAIDS); and Robert Crown, World Bank (Ret.). Charles Griffin, HNP Sector Manager, and Girindre Beeharry, Health Economist, LCSHD, Latin America and Caribbean Region, World Bank, contributed the section on cost simulations for HIV/AIDS programs in the Caribbean, on the basis of a simulation exercise done in conjunction with the Caribbean Epidemiology Center (CAREC), the Pan American Health Organization/World Health Organization (PAHO/WHO), University of West Indies (UWI), and the World Bank. The report benefited from information, detailed comments and advice provided by Peggy McEvoy, UNAIDS Team Leader for the Caribbean; and Barrington Wint, Health Manager, Caribbean Community (CARICOM). Lani Rice Marquez, University Research Co., LLC, reviewed the draft version and provided insightful comments and advice. Kerry B. Kemp, Aracelly Woodall, Maria Colchao and Patricia Bernedo edited and supported the production of the report, respectively.

Valuable comments and suggestions were provided on various drafts by Debrework Zewdie (Global HIV/AIDS Coordinator for the World Bank); Christopher Lovelace (Director, Health, Nutrition and Population-HDNHE-, World Bank); Charles Griffin (HNP Sector Manager, LCSHD, World Bank); William Experton (HD Sector Leader, LCC3C, World Bank); Anabela Abreu (LCSHD, World Bank); Tressa Alfred (World Bank); Florence Baingana (HDNHE, World Bank); Girindre Beeharry (LCSHD, World Bank); Paloma Cuchi PAHO/WHO); Maria Donoso-Clark (LCC3C, World Bank); Oscar Echeverri (Public Health Specialist, Cali, Colombia); Michele Gragnolati (LCSHD, World Bank); Ruth Levine (LCSHD, World Bank); Miguel A. Marquez (Special Adviser, UNDP); Sandra Rosenhouse (LCSHD, World Bank); Miriam Schneidman (LCSHD, World Bank); Diana Weil (HDNHE, WHO/World Bank); and Fernando Zacarias (PAHO/WHO).

The report draws heavily from data and assessments on the HIV/AIDS pandemic prepared by UNAIDS, CARICOM, CAREC, PAHO/WHO, and the World Bank.

The report was prepared in the Human Development Sector Management Unit, Latin America and Caribbean Region, at the request of the Caribbean Country Management Unit, Latin America and Caribbean Region, under the leadership of Xavier Coll (Director) and Orsalia Kalantzopoulos (Director), respectively.

The report was presented during the Meeting of the Caribbean Group on Cooperation in Economic Development (CGCED)," held at the World Bank June 12-16, 2000. This meeting involved Prime Ministers, Ministers of Finance and other key decision-makers from member countries, country delegations as well as senior representatives of other international organizations, who assigned the highest priority to deal with the HIV/AIDS epidemic in the region.

The report was further disseminated during the Regional Conference on HIV/AIDS held in Barbados, September 11-12, 2000. The Government of Barbados, together with the CARICOM Secretariat, PAHO/WHO, UNAIDS and the World Bank sponsored the Conference. Present at the Conference were Prime Ministers of Barbados, the Bahamas, St Vincent and the Grenadines and St Kitts and Navis, the Chief Minister of Anguilla, as well as ministers of health, population and/or social development from The Bahamas (also represented by the Minister of Finance), Barbados (represented by Cabinet), Belize, Cuba, Dominica, Grenada, Haiti, Jamaica, St Kitts and Nevis, St Lucia, Trinidad and Tobago, Turks and Caicos, representatives of the Presidential Commission on HIV/AIDS from the Dominican Republic as well as high level representatives from Antigua & Barbuda, Aruba, Guyana, Montserrat and Suriname. Representatives of major bilateral and multilateral agencies active in the Caribbean, and representatives of civil society, academia and the media also participated.

ACRONYMS AND ABBREVIATIONS

AIDS	Acquired Immunodeficiency Syndrome
AIDSCAP	AIDS Control and Prevention Project
APL	Adaptable Program Lending
ARV	Antiretroviral
AZT	Azidothymidine (now called zidovudine)
CAREC	Caribbean Epidemiology Center
CARICOM	Caribbean Community and Common Market
CARIFORUM	Caribbean Forum
CAS	Country Assistance Strategy
CHHP	Caribbean Healthy Hotels Project
CIDA	Canadian International Development Agency
CSW	Commercial Sex Workers
CRN+	Caribbean Network of People Living with HIV/AIDS
DFID	British Department for International Development
GTZ	German Technical Cooperation
CTO	Caribbean Tourism Organization
DOTS	Directly Observed Treatment, Short course (for tuberculosis)
EDF	Economic Development Fund
EU	European Union
FTC	French Technical Cooperation
GAVI	Global Alliance for Vaccines and Immunizations
GDP	Gross Domestic Product
HAART	Highly Active Anti-Retroviral Therapy
HFLE	Health and Family Life Education Program
HIV	Human Immunodeficiency Virus
IADB	Inter-American Development Bank
IAVI	International AIDS Vaccine Initiative
IDU	Injecting Drug Use
IEC	Information, Education, and Communication
IFC	International Finance Corporation
IMF	International Monetary Fund
IMPACT	Implementing AIDS Care and Prevention Project
MSM	Men who have Sex with Men
NGO	Nongovernmental Organizations
OECS	Organization of Eastern Caribbean States
PAHO	Pan American Health Organization
PROMESS	Programme des Medicaments Essentiels (Essential Drugs Program) (Haiti)
SIDALAC	Regional AIDS Initiative for Latin America and the Caribbean
STD/I	Sexually Transmitted Disease/Infections
TB	Tuberculosis
UNAIDS	Joint United Nations Program on HIV/AIDS
UNDCP	United Nations International Drug Control Programme
UNDP	United Nations Development Programme
UNESCO	United Nations Educational, Scientific, and Cultural Organization
UNFPA	United Nations Fund for Population Activities
UNICEF	United Nations Children's Fund
USAID	United States Agency for International Development
UWI	University of West Indies
WHO	World Health Organization

Official estimates—which are undoubtedly low—indicate that 360,000 people are living with HIV/AIDS[1] in the Caribbean region and that the percentage of adults ages 15 to 49 living with HIV/AIDS is approaching 2%. However, given widespread underreporting in the region, it is estimated that more than half a million people are infected with HIV. Out of the twelve countries with the highest HIV prevalence in Latin America and the Caribbean region, nine are in the Caribbean. In Haiti, the Bahamas, Barbados, the Dominican Republic, and Guyana, the HIV/AIDS epidemic has spread to the general population. In other Caribbean countries, the HIV/AIDS epidemic is still concentrated among the population groups who engage in high-risk behavior[2]—commercial sex workers, men who have sex with men, and injecting drug users—but it is accelerating rapidly and is posed to strike the general population. Currently, the primary mode of transmission of HIV/AIDS in the Caribbean is sexual intercourse between men and women. Women now account for more than a third of all AIDS cases in the Caribbean, and the infants of HIV-infected mothers can contract the disease during pregnancy, childbirth, or breast-feeding. Many young people begin sexual intercourse at an early age in the Caribbean, and since they tend not to use condoms to protect themselves, they are at high risk of contracting HIV.

Intensified efforts are needed in the Caribbean region if inroads are to be made against the AIDS epidemic. Although many Caribbean governments have initiated a limited response to HIV/AIDS, much remains to be done to bring proven interventions quickly up to nationwide scale. There is no time to delay because HIV/AIDS is unique among diseases in combining seven attributes:

- HIV spreads very fast.

- People who contract HIV may remain infectious for many years without knowing they have the virus or showing any symptoms. The potential for spread is high.

- It reduces life expectancy, which is positively related to savings, productivity, and education.

- HIV/AIDS primarily affects young people, ages 15 to 49, who are in the prime of their lives as workers and parents.

- People with AIDS suffer repeated and prolonged illnesses, imposing great costs on households and health systems.

- AIDS breaks down social cohesion, challenges value systems, and raises deeply rooted and sensitive gender inequalities.

- There is no AIDS vaccine and no cure.

There is a growing recognition that HIV/AIDS is not just a serious health issue in developing countries, but a major developmental catastrophe that threatens to dismantle the social and economic achievements of the past half century. The challenge for Caribbean countries is to

---

1 AIDS stands for "acquired immunodeficiency syndrome" (a syndrome being a cluster of medical conditions). AIDS is caused by the human immunodeficiency virus (HIV), which weakens and then destroys the body's immune system, leaving a person vulnerable to serious "opportunistic infections" (e.g., tuberculosis, pneumonia) which ultimately lead to death.

2 High-risk behavior is defined as engaging in unprotected (i.e., without a condom) sexual intercourse with many partners or sharing of unsterilized needles or other injecting equipment.

learn from the dramatic experiences of some African countries and act decisively now to prevent the progressive extension of the epidemic to the general population. What happened in Africa in less than two decades could now happen in the Caribbean if action is not taken while the epidemic is in the early stages. Fortunately, there is still an opportunity in the Caribbean to prevent HIV/AIDS rates from escalating to the alarming levels found in many sub-Saharan African countries.

This report provides an overview of the challenges and opportunities in addressing the problem of HIV/AIDS in the Caribbean. It presents a snapshot the HIV/AIDS epidemic in the region, offers examples of ways in which Caribbean countries and regional bodies such as the Caribbean Community (CARICOM) have responded to the epidemic, discuss alternative actions for addressing the crisis, and highlights a range of strategies for donor coordination and cooperation in the region. Finally, the report identifies the potential role of the World Bank in addressing the HIV/AIDS epidemic in the Caribbean.

THE SPREAD OF HIV/AIDS IN THE CARIBBEAN

Prevalence of HIV in the Caribbean

With the HIV prevalence among Caribbean adults ages 15 to 49 approaching 2%, the *Caribbean region currently has the highest HIV prevalence rate of any region in the world other than the AIDS-ravaged sub-Saharan Africa,* where the prevalence of HIV among adults ages 15 to 49 is reported to be 8.0%.

As noted below, the primary reported mode of HIV transmission among adults in the Caribbean region is sexual intercourse between men and women. In part because women are more vulnerable to HIV infection than men due to gender inequality issues, the percentage of women with the disease is rising. As of 1999, about 35% of the adults affected with HIV in the Caribbean region were women.

Mother-to-child or vertical transmission now accounts for 6% of all reported AIDS cases in the Caribbean region.

Incidence of AIDS in the Caribbean

CARICOM estimates that more new cases of HIV/AIDS were reported in the Caribbean between 1995 and 1998 than had been reported since the beginning of the epidemic in the early 1980s. Currently, *the Caribbean region has the highest AIDS incidence rate—i.e., number of new AIDS cases per million population per year—in the Americas.* From 1991 to 1996, the AIDS incidence rate in the English-speaking Caribbean increased from 142.3 new AIDS per million to 246.2 cases per million. In the Latin Caribbean countries, although Cuba remains with a low AIDS incidence rate, data from Haiti and the Dominican Republic show a similar upward trend. If Puerto Rico is included in the Latin Caribbean figures, the observed trend becomes more pronounced.

Modes of HIV Transmission in the Caribbean

The primary mode of HIV transmission in the Caribbean is *unprotected sexual intercourse—that is, sexual intercourse without use of a condom.* More than half of all the AIDS reported cases in the Caribbean region are the result of unprotected sexual intercourse between men and women.

Apart from sexual transmission, other modes of HIV transmission in the Caribbean region are the use of contaminated needles by intravenous drug users; blood-borne transmission; and, increasingly, mother-to-child perinatal transmission.

Mortality and Socioeconomic Impacts of HIV/AIDS in the Caribbean

In the English-speaking Caribbean, AIDS is now the largest cause of death among young men between the ages of 15 and 44. In some parts of the Dominican Republic, AIDS has become the most common cause of death among young women, in particular, women between 20 and 34 years of age. By the end of 1999, the cumulative number of Caribbean children estimated to have been orphaned by HIV/AIDS at age 14 or younger stood at 83,000. The emergence of AIDS as a major health problem places a tremendous burden on the health care systems of the Caribbean countries. HIV has a long latency period, so some of the social and economic consequences of the HIV/AIDS epidemic may not be felt immediately. Eventually, however, unless the epidemic is curbed, economic sectors such as agriculture, tourism, mining, lumber, finance, and trade will suffer as a result of lost productivity due to AIDS-related illness and premature deaths among economically active adults.

As recognized by the United Nations Security Council, and the United States Government, HIV/AIDS has manifested itself as not only a challenge to sustainable development but has now become a threat to national sovereignty and global security. These concerns are highly relevant for the Caribbean because its HIV/AIDS epidemic could create significant externalities beyond the region (e.g., according to recent health data, the fastest growing epidemic within Canada is amongst Canadians from the Caribbean, mainly Haitian in Montreal; the second highest urban HIV seroprevalence in the United States is found in San Juan, Puerto Rico). The high-profile international attention to this issue implies that Caribbean governments cannot deny or ignore it anymore.

INTENSIFYING ACTION AGAINST HIV/AIDS: KEY CHALLENGES FOR CARIBBEAN COUNTRIES

Prevention of HIV/AIDS in Caribbean Countries

In order to be successful, HIV/AIDS prevention campaigns in Caribbean countries must work on three basic levels:

- *Preventing the sexual transmission of HIV in young people and adults.* Young people represent half of the people who become infected with HIV. For that reason, great importance needs to be given to ensure sure that young people, along with the adult population, have understanding, motivation, skills, tools, and freedom to adopt behaviors that protect them from HIV infection. Reaching young people is a key element in the prevention of the AIDS epidemic.

- *Preventing mother-to-child transmission of HIV.* Many HIV-positive women in developing countries, including the Caribbean, do not have access to prophylactic drugs that can help prevent HIV transmission during pregnancy and delivery. Furthermore, HIV-positive women in developing countries breast-feed their babies and transmit HIV to them that way. Nevirapine (sold as Viramune) appears to prevent mother-to-child HIV transmission even better than the antiviral drug zidovudine (AZT) and at a considerably lower cost. Information gaps need to be addressed in order to make final recommendations on breast-feeding and medical care policies for HIV-positive women in Caribbean countries.

- *Preventing blood-borne transmission of HIV.* The screening of donated blood and plasma for HIV antibody began in the Caribbean in 1985. People at risk have also been encouraged not to donate blood. The fact that transmission of HIV through blood or blood products accounts for less than 3% of AIDS cases in most of the Caribbean suggests that additional efforts are needed to eliminate this source of infection.

Diagnosis of HIV/AIDS in Caribbean Countries

HIV testing is available in both public and private sector laboratories in the Caribbean. In Caribbean Epidemiology Center (CAREC) member countries, total requests for HIV testing in public sector laboratories rose 44% from 1986 and 1994, and recent trends indicate that the demand for testing will continue to increase.

Care and Treatment of People with HIV/AIDS in Caribbean Countries

The treatment of HIV/AIDS in most Caribbean countries, as in other developing countries, is negligible. Public health programs are under-funded in some countries that health agencies cannot afford inexpensive medications for opportunistic infections such as tuberculosis, much less the thousands of dollars it can cost to treat a single patient with the new combinations of antiviral drugs. In several countries, religious institutions and nongovernmental organizations (NGOs) are the primary providers of care for people living with HIV/AIDS. Their efforts have expanded partly in response to the growing deficiencies in HIV/AIDS care offered by the public health sector. A representative of the Caribbean Network for People Living with HIV/AIDS (CRN+) notes that an HIV-positive diagnosis is usually seen as a death sentence in the Caribbean. People suspected of being HIV-positive are scorned and cast out. The wider community needs more education to combat this stigmatization and discrimination.

Prospects for the Development of an AIDS Vaccine

There is no certainty that a vaccine which will be suitable, effective, and affordable in developing countries will be developed in the foreseeable future. Just as the hope for improved access to costly AIDS drugs should not undermine a strong and unrelenting effort to prevent HIV transmission in developing countries through existing preventive measures, neither should the hope of an AIDS vaccine.

Intensifying National Responses to HIV/AIDS in the Caribbean: Five Key Steps

Governments of all Caribbean countries (with their development partners) need to expand and intensify their responses rapidly, and to address HIV/AIDS as a multisectoral development issue—not only a health concern. At the national level, the following five actions are fundamental:

- *Step #1: Increase the national government's commitment, attention, and funding to combat the HIV/AIDS epidemic.* It is vital that national leaders in the Caribbean region turn their full attention to the challenges of the epidemic. Their support is crucial to the long-term success of any national or regional effort.

- *Step #2: Scale up HIV/AIDS prevention activities at the national and community levels.* In scaling up HIV/AIDS prevention activities, the focus in Caribbean countries should be on a core set of prevention activities already shown to be both effective and feasible: (1) communications that move audiences, especially youths, from awareness of HIV/AIDS to risk-reducing behavior; (2) making condoms, the treatment of STDs, and voluntary counseling and testing for HIV more accessible; (3) ensuring a safe blood supply; and (4) reducing mother-to-child transmission of HIV. Communities and NGOs should receive direct financial support for prevention activities at the local level.

- *Step #3: Scale up HIV/AIDS care activities at the national and community levels.* Strategies should be mounted by Caribbean countries and their partners to provide high-quality community and home-based care to people with HIV/AIDS. Also needed are programs to care for the children orphaned by AIDS.

- *Step #4: Support more HIV/AIDS-related research at the national level.* Continued research is needed into the cost of HIV/AIDS treatment and care alternatives, impact and costs of HIV/AIDS for different economic sectors, and the effectiveness of existing tools in different cultural and infrastructure settings.

- *Step #5: Strengthen regional responses to the epidemic in the Caribbean.* Regional responses to the HIV/AIDS epidemic are discussed below.

REGIONAL RESPONSES TO HIV/AIDS IN THE CARIBBEAN

There are several good arguments for mounting a strong regional response to HIV/AIDS in the Caribbean region. First, most of the countries in the Caribbean region are too small and/or too poor to support a national capacity to respond adequately to the HIV/AIDS epidemic. Second, with migration, the HIV/AID epidemic is clearly a problem that transcends national boundaries. International donors could assist Caribbean countries and regional organizations in their efforts to mount an effective regional response to the epidemic.

The Response of the Caribbean Countries

All of the Caribbean countries have established National AIDS Programs and developed short- and medium-term plans for responding to the epidemic. Caribbean governments—in partnership with regional and international agencies—have sought to address the various aspects of the epidemic in the region. As a result, throughout the Caribbean region, there are country-level successes. Yet, despite these efforts, what is needed in most of the Caribbean countries is a comprehensive, multisectoral national response that engages government, civil society, and international donors, as well as scaled up efforts to serve entire national populations.

International Donors' Activities Related to HIV/AIDS in the Caribbean

The European Union (EU) and its member countries, the Joint United Nations Program on AIDS (UNAIDS) and its co-sponsors, the U.S. Agency for International Development (USAID), and the Canadian International Development Agency (CIDA) are the primary international donors involved in the HIV/AIDS-related activities in Caribbean countries. Currently, the EU and its member states are the major external financiers of the response to HIV/AIDS in the Caribbean, having committed or disbursed over 11 million Euros to date. The EU is contemplating a major new initiative to assist CARICOM member states respond to HIV/AIDS: *Strengthening the Institutional Response to HIV/AIDS in the Caribbean Project.* However, the proposed project, which will last three years and cost 6.425 million Euros, is not yet effective. It involves six regional agencies: CARICOM, CAREC, CRN+, UNAIDS, the Caribbean Research Council and the University of the West Indies.

Caribbean Regional Organizations' HIV/AIDS-Related Initiatives

The Secretariat of the CARICOM—the organization responsible for regional policy and cooperation in the Caribbean region—has assumed a lead role in regional HIV/AIDS initiatives in the Caribbean. The Caribbean Task Force on HIV/AIDS, chaired by the CARICOM Secretariat, recently led a wide consultation process and developed a comprehensive five-year strategic plan for the region. That plan is discussed further below.

Two other organizations involved in regional HIV/AIDS initiatives in the Caribbean are CAREC and the CRN+. CAREC operates a Special Program on Sexually Transmitted Infections in the English- and Dutch-speaking Caribbean countries. CRN+, an organization established in 1996, is based in Trinidad and Tobago but has affiliates in 17 countries in the region. Its goals are to share information, build capacity among persons living with HIV/AIDS, and support HIV/AIDS advocacy efforts in the Caribbean.

The Caribbean Regional Strategic Plan of Action for HIV/AIDS

The *Caribbean Regional Strategic Plan of Action for HIV/AIDS, 1999-2004,* includes six major areas for regional action: (1) advocacy, policy development, and legislation; (2) care and support of people living with HIV/AIDS; (3) prevention of HIV transmission in young people; (4) prevention of HIV transmission among vulnerable populations; (5) prevention of mother-to-child transmission of HIV; and (6) strengthening national and regional response capabilities. The National AIDS Program Directors met in Antigua in June 1999 to review and approve the draft regional strategic plan, and the final version of the plan was published in February 2000. The implementation of the five-year plan will be overseen by the Caribbean Task Force on HIV/AIDS under CARICOM's leadership. The activities called for in the plan will be financed largely through existing and new programs and projects. The success of this CARICOM-led regional effort will hinge on the willingness of the leaders of the Caribbean countries to collaborate, as well as on the commitment of the EU, the World Bank, and other international donors.

THE WORLD BANK'S ROLE IN THE CARIBBEAN

What Has Been Done by the World Bank?

The World Bank is one the leading financiers of HIV/AIDS activities in the world. Since 1986, the Bank has committed over US$988.5 million worldwide to more than 80 ongoing and future projects to prevent and control the spread of HIV/AIDS. In sub-Saharan Africa, the World Bank has recently adopted a new strategic approach to addressing the devastating consequences of HIV/AIDS on development. In the new strategy, the World Bank treats AIDS as a priority development issue that impacts upon all sectors of the economy and focuses on bringing successful interventions to a national or regional scale.

What Could Be Done by the World Bank in the Caribbean?

Except in the Dominican Republic and Haiti, the World Bank's presence in the health sector of the wider Caribbean is relatively limited. The World Bank could broaden its activities in the Caribbean to have a significant impact on the HIV/AIDS epidemic there (1) by actively participating in UNAIDS and local U.N. Theme Groups on HIV/AIDS; and (2) by incorporating

HIV/AIDS prevention and control activities for Caribbean countries into its country assistance strategies and lending programs.

Operationalizing an HIV/AIDS Prevention and Control Strategy in the Caribbean

The World Bank could finance a Multi-Country HIV/AIDS Adaptable Program Lending (APL) for the Caribbean to assist the governments of the region to scale up HIV/AIDS prevention and control activities. It would help build strong regional and national leadership with broad participation, and establish an institutional platform for long-term sustainability. In coordination with the International Finance Corporation (IFC) efforts could also be made to enlist the private sector in HIV/AIDS prevention and control efforts. Additionally, as done in Brazil, World Bank support may help promote active involvement of civil society organizations. According to recent estimates about US$260 million per year, or a 10-fold increase in current national, international and private spending on HIV/AIDS prevention and care, would be needed to effectively slow the spread of HIV and to treat AIDS victims with dignity and compassion.

Conclusion

No single step will suffice to curb the relentless spread of the HIV/AIDS epidemic in the countries of the Caribbean. What is needed is a balanced combination of advocacy, incentives, disincentives, funding, and policy support. *The overarching goal of support for developing countries from the World Bank and other development partners should be to help every country at risk to establish an appropriate national HIV/AIDS program comprising basic prevention, basic treatment, and basic care. It should be clear, however, that while costly drugs are available to a small percentage of the world's people, behavior change is the only way to safeguard against infection in most of the world.* Concerted action by Caribbean governments and Caribbean regional agencies such as CARICOM, in partnership with civil society, the private sector and NGOs, and with the assistance of the international community, will help to mitigate the adverse impact of AIDS on people of the Caribbean region in years to come.

"Many of us used to think of AIDS as a health issue. We were wrong. AIDS can no longer be confined to the health or social sector portfolios. AIDS is turning back the clock on development."

James Wolfensohn, "War on AIDS," Appearance by World Bank President before U.N. Security Council, January 10, 2000.

I INTRODUCTION

THE HIV/AIDS GLOBAL EPIDEMIC

As reported in newspaper articles and other publications, a deadly scourge lies beneath the "tropical tranquility" of the Caribbean—HIV/AIDS. AIDS stands for "acquired immunodeficiency syndrome" (a syndrome being a cluster of medical conditions). AIDS is caused by the human immunodeficiency virus (HIV), which weakens and then destroys the body's immune system. HIV/AIDS has spread rapidly in the last two decades, causing massive human death and suffering, particularly in the developing world. There is a growing recognition that HIV/AIDS is not just a serious health issue in developing countries, but a major developmental catastrophe that threatens to dismantle the social and economic achievements of the past half-century.

What is HIV/AIDS and How Does it Spread?

HIV/AIDS is a fatal, sexually transmitted disease or infection (STD). Once a person is infected with HIV, he or she is infected for life. In all but a very small proportion of cases, HIV/AIDS destroys a person's immune system. The time between becoming HIV positive and the onset of AIDS varies. In industrialized countries, the average time between infection with HIV and the appearance of symptoms is about 10 years, but in the poorest countries of the world, without access to proper care, the time is sometimes as short as five years. Once an HIV-infected person's immune system is severely damaged, he or she becomes vulnerable to life-threatening "opportunistic infections" (e.g., pneumonia, tuberculosis) and is diagnosed as having AIDS. Most patients succumb to opportunistic infections within two years after the onset of AIDS (UNAIDS, 1999).

Worldwide, about half of all of the people who become infected with HIV acquire the infection before age 25, and they typically die of the opportunistic affections associated with AIDS before their 35th birthday. For this reason, AIDS is uniquely threatening to both young people who are at risk for infection and children who are orphaned by HIV/AIDS. According to UNAIDS, the Joint United Nations Program on AIDS, by the end of 1999, the AIDS epidemic had left behind a cumulative total of 11.2 million orphans, defined as children having lost their mother before reaching the age of 15 (UNAIDS, 1999).

Not everybody is equally likely to become infected with HIV and to transmit it to others. Like other STDs, HIV is difficult to spread except by sex or other direct contact with the bodily fluids of an infected person (see Box 1-1). About three-quarters of HIV transmission worldwide occurs through sexual intercourse; of these cases, about three-quarters involve heterosexual intercourse and one-quarter involve sexual relations between men. The other modes of HIV transmission are transfusions of contaminated blood or blood products, reuse of contaminated syringes by injecting drug users, infection via birth or nursing from an HIV-positive mother to her child during pregnancy, childbirth, or breast-feeding, and reuse of needles in medical settings. HIV cannot be transmitted by a sneeze, a handshake, or other casual contact (Confronting AIDS, 1998).

In the United States and other industrialized countries, medical breakthroughs have prolonged and improved the quality of lives of people living with HIV. As noted in a recent World Bank publication, however, medical breakthroughs in treating HIV infection in industrialized countries, although encouraging, are still very far from offering a technologically feasible or affordable cure for the people in the developing world (Confronting AIDS, 1998).

HIV/AIDS: A Still-Emerging Epidemic

The extent of the global HIV/AIDS epidemic is suggested by the numbers presented in Table 1-1. By the end of 1999, 33.6 million people worldwide were living with HIV, including 1.2 million children under the age of 15. About 95% of these 33.6 million HIV-positive people resided in developing countries. The countries of the developing world have also experienced 95% of all deaths to date from AIDS, largely among young adults in their peak productive and reproductive years. In some countries of sub-Saharan Africa, the social, economic, and other effects of AIDS deaths have already reached crisis levels. The impacts in other countries will be magnified as HIV infection rates continue to rise, particularly in countries where

---

Box 1-1. Facts About AIDS

- Human immunodeficiency virus (HIV) is a "retrovirus" that spreads through unprotected sexual intercourse (that is, intercourse without a condom), transfusions of unscreened blood contaminated with HIV, needles contaminated with HIV (most frequently for injecting drug use but also in medical settings), and from infected women to their child during pregnancy, childbirth, or breast-feeding.

- HIV is a slow-acting virus. The majority of HIV-infected individuals look healthy and feel well for many years after infection; they may not even suspect they harbor the virus, though they can transmit it to others. It is estimated that 90% of all HIV-infected people worldwide do not know they have the virus. A laboratory blood or saliva test is the only certain way to determine whether an individual is HIV-positive.

- Once an individual has an established HIV infection, he or she is infected for life. HIV weakens a person's immune system, reducing the person's ability to fight off illnesses. As the immune system loses its ability to fight off infections, serious illnesses, called "opportunistic infections," appear. Treatment with antiretroviral (ARV) drugs can slow the progression of HIV infection to the serious illnesses that define AIDS, but these expensive medications are not available to most people in the developing world, who often lack access even to drugs that combat opportunistic infections. Thus, most people in the developing world succumb to serious opportunistic infections within two years after the onset of AIDS.

Source: UNAIDS, 1999.

---

poverty, poor health systems, and limited resources for prevention and care fuel the spread of HIV. In most developing countries, treatment of HIV/AIDS is negligible, and health systems are struggling even to provide symptomatic care or the treatment of opportunistic infections among people with HIV/AIDS.

Table 1-1. Global Summary of the HIV/AIDS Epidemic, December 1999		
People newly infected with HIV in 1999	**TOTAL** Adults *Women* Children < 15 years	**5.6 million** 5 million *2.3 million* 570,000
Number of people living with HIV/AIDS	**TOTAL** Adults *Women* Children < 15 years	**33.6 million** 32.4 million *14.8 million* 1.2 million
AIDS deaths in 1999	**TOTAL** Adults *Women* Children < 15 years	**2.6 million** 2.1 million *1.1 million* 470,000
Total number of AIDS deaths since the beginning of the epidemic	**TOTAL** Adults *Women* Children < 15 years	**16.3 million** 12.7 million *6.2 million* 3.6 million

Source: UNAIDS, 1999.

Impacts of the Disease

HIV/AIDS is unique among diseases in combining seven attributes:[3]

- HIV spreads very fast.

- People who contract HIV may remain infectious for many years without knowing they have the virus or showing any symptoms. The potential for spread is high.

- It reduces life expectancy, which is positively related to savings, productivity, and education.

- HIV/AIDS primarily affects young people, ages 15 to 49, who are in the prime of their lives as workers and parents.

- People with AIDS suffer repeated and prolonged illnesses, imposing great costs on households and health systems.

- AIDS breaks down social cohesion, challenges value systems, and raises deeply rooted and sensitive gender inequalities.

- There is no AIDS vaccine and no cure.

In some parts of Africa, HIV/AIDS is already reversing hard-won gains in life expectancy made during the last four decades. Average life expectancy in developing countries rose from 49 years in 1950 to 70 years in 1990. In southern Africa, life expectancy at birth rose from 44 years in the early 1950s to 59 in the early 1990s; as a result of AIDS, however, life

---

3 This section is largely from the World Bank's document "Intensifying Action Against HIV/AIDS," presented to the Development Committee, April 17, 2000.

expectancy in the region is now set to drop back to 45 years between 2005 and 2010. In contrast, people living in south Asia, who could barely expect to reach their 40th birthday in 1950, can expect by 2005 to be living 22 years longer than their counterparts in AIDS-ravaged southern Africa (UNAIDS, 1999). This too, however, will be challenged unless the Asian sub-epidemic is confronted vigorously before it reaches African dimensions.

As the number of HIV/AIDS rises in a developing country or region, the negative consequences become more severe. Health systems become overburdened. The fiscal cost of HIV/AIDS is significant. One year of basic treatment for a person with AIDS costs an estimated two to three times the per capita gross domestic product (GDP) in medical costs alone. Most of these costs are typically borne by the public sector, which faces difficult choices. As the number of AIDS cases increases, so does the cost. In a country with HIV prevalence of 15% (i.e., 15% of the population is infected with the virus), the estimated budgetary cost could rise from 2.5% of GDP today to 6.0% by 2010. In sub-Saharan Africa, there is massive suffering due to HIV/AIDS, and millions of children have been orphaned by the disease. Social systems have become overburdened, and the health and education gains of the poor have been reversed.

Recent World Bank research suggests that HIV/AIDS has a substantial negative impact on economic growth. This relationship was difficult to discern when HIV prevalence rates were lower, but it now appears that the economic impact grows as the HIV/AIDS epidemic advances. As long as prevalence of HIV remains below about 5%, per capita growth is minimally affected. As prevalence rises, per capita growth begins to decline, as shown in Figure 1-1. When the prevalence reaches 8%—about where it is in 21 African countries today—the cost in per capita growth is about 0.4 percentage points per year. Compared to historical performance in Africa, such losses are significant. Annual per capita growth in

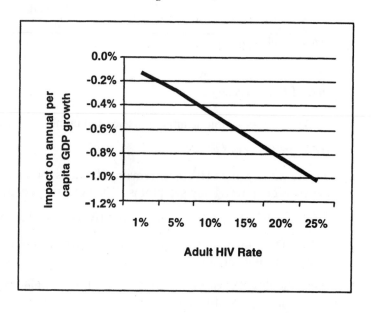

Figure 1-1. Estimated Impact of AIDS on per Capita Growth

Africa as a whole for the past three years has been about 1.2%, for instance. In countries such as Zimbabwe, where the HIV prevalence rate exceeds 25%, annual per capita growth is probably a full percentage point lower than it otherwise would be.

THE CHALLENGE OF RESPONDING TO HIV/AIDS[4]

If action is not taken while the epidemic is young, what happened in Africa in less than two decades could now happen anywhere in developing and transition economies. Although the spread of HIV infection is largely the result of private decisions, government intervention to prevent it is justified for several reasons:

- As recognized by the United Nations Security Council and the United States Government, HIV/AIDS has manifested itself as not only a challenge to sustainable development but has now become a threat to national sovereignty and global security.

- Some individuals cannot control their own risk of HIV infection (e.g., spouses, newborns, victims of rape, accident victims who need a blood transfusion).

- Information regarding HIV transmission is imperfect.

- HIV makes people vulnerable to other infectious diseases, including tuberculosis.

- AIDS cannot be cured.

- Adult deaths impose costs on other family members and the rest of society.

- AIDS may increase both the magnitude and depth of poverty.

- Markets to insure against premature deaths and HIV are incomplete.

In the Caribbean region and elsewhere, many national governments have initiated a response to HIV/AIDS. Few, however, have brought their response to the scale necessary. More than 360,000 people are reported living with HIV/AIDS in the wider, independent Caribbean, and the percentage of adults ages 15 to 49 living with AIDS is 2%. The HIV/AIDS epidemic in the Caribbean is second only to that of sub-Saharan Africa in terms of its percentage of adult population affected and rate of acceleration. In some Caribbean countries (the Bahamas, Barbados, the Dominican Republic, Guyana, Haiti) HIV/AIDS epidemic has already spread to the general population. Some of these countries (e.g., Haiti) have some of the poorest socio-economic and health indicators in the Western Hemisphere, which will only exacerbate the HIV/AIDS problem. In other Caribbean countries, while the HIV/AIDS epidemic is largely concentrated among certain population groups practicing high-risk behaviors (e.g., commercial sex workers, men having sex with men), it is accelerating rapidly and is posed to spread to the rest of the population. Puerto Rico, a Caribbean island that is geographically and functionally central to the region, has the second highest urban HIV infection rate within the United States. Though officially included within United States statistics, Puerto Rico must be considered when estimating the true impact of the epidemic upon Caribbean peoples and resources. The challenge for these countries, therefore, is to learn from the experiences of some African countries and act decisively now to prevent the progressive extension of the epidemic from these groups to the rest of the population. Multisectoral and multidisciplinary development approaches are therefore needed to intervene effectively and address vulnerability in a broader environment where situations of risk occur.

---

4 This section is based on the World Bank's document "Intensifying Action Against HIV/AIDS," presented to the Development Committee, April 17, 2000. It also draws from another World Bank document: "Confronting AIDS," 1998.

There is now growing support for the rapid intensification of international action against HIV/AIDS. Ministers attending the 61st meeting of the Development Committee of the World Bank/International Monetary Fund (IMF) held in Washington, DC, on April 17, 2000, for example, recognized that the HIV/AIDS epidemic not only poses an acute danger to development in sub-Saharan Africa, but is also a rapidly growing threat in Asia and the Caribbean, and a probable threat in many Eastern European countries and elsewhere as well (see Box 1-2). Clearly, the governments of developing countries cannot address the HIV/AIDS problem alone. Given the scope of the epidemic and limited resources of these countries, sustained support from the World Bank and other development partners of these countries will be required. The overriding goal of support in the Caribbean region should be to help every country at risk develop an appropriate national HIV/AIDS program comprising basic prevention, basic treatment, and basic care.

Box 1-2. Communiqué of the 61ˢᵗ Meeting of the Development Committee of the World Bank/IMF on Intensifying Action Against HIV/AIDS, April 17, 2000

Ministers at the meeting emphasized that the HIV/AIDS epidemic, which has already infected about 50 million people worldwide, is not only a very serious public health concern and the cause of great human suffering, but a severe danger to development progress itself. Ministers recognized that HIV/AIDS weakens economic growth, governance, human capital, labor productivity, and the investment climate, thereby undermining the foundations of development and poverty reduction. Ministers noted that the epidemic now not only poses an acute danger to development in sub-Saharan Africa, but is a rapidly growing threat in Asia and the Caribbean, and a probable threat in many Eastern European countries and elsewhere as well. As HIV spreads quickly, even countries with currently low infection rates cannot afford to delay strengthening anti-HIV/AIDS programs.

In view of this alarming situation, the Committee called for rapid intensification of international action on the global HIV/AIDS crisis. Given the urgency of prevention and the vast needs for care and treatment, the Committee stressed the importance of effective partnerships to encourage each actor in the international system to focus on its comparative strength. Ministers urged governments, international agencies, civil society, the media and the private sector, including the pharmaceutical industry, to step up their efforts, building on experience gained in ongoing activities. They urged developing and transition countries to increase their political and economic commitment to combating HIV/AIDS, to address the epidemic on a multisectoral basis, to scale up programs to nationwide—and in some cases, regional—scope, to strengthen the primary health care systems needed for effective delivery of services, and to provide more resources directly to local communities. The Committee encouraged industrialized countries and international organizations to mainstream HIV/AIDS in their development programs and to devote increased financial and institutional resources on a scale commensurate with the scope of the crisis. Ministers recognized that support for capacity building is particularly important in addressing this long-lasting development problem.

Ministers welcomed the World Bank's expanded efforts against HIV/AIDS, in particular its active participation in the UNAIDS partnership, its new HIV/AIDS strategy for Africa, and its work with the Global Alliance for Vaccines and Immunizations. They urged the Bank to intensify its HIV/AIDS work on a global basis, focusing on its areas of expertise, and called on the World Bank and the IMF to take full account of HIV/AIDS in their support for poverty reduction strategies and the HIPC (Heavily Indebted Poor Countries) Initiative.

Source: World Bank, 2000.

REPORT OBJECTIVES

This report provides an overview of the challenges and opportunities in addressing the problem of HIV/AIDS in the Caribbean. The following chapters present information concerning selected HIV/AIDS topics relevant to the Caribbean, attempt to capture the state of HIV/AIDS in the region as it moves into the 21st Century, offer examples of ways in which the countries of the Caribbean have responded to the mosaic of HIV/AIDS epidemics in the region, discuss alternative actions for addressing the crisis, and highlight a range of strategies for donor coordination and cooperation in the region, including the World Bank. The report draws heavily from data and assessments prepared by UNAIDS, the Caribbean Community (CARICOM), the Caribbean Epidemiology Center (CAREC), the Pan American Health Organization/World Health Organization (PAHO/WHO), and World Bank documents.

"AIDS is far more than a medical problem. AIDS is far more than a national problem. AIDS is far from over."

Kofi A. Annan, Secretary-General of the United Nations.

II THE SPREAD OF HIV/AIDS IN THE CARIBBEAN

THE CARIBBEAN: A HETEROGENEOUS REGION

The Caribbean region is an extraordinarily diverse region of about 36 million people (see Box 2-1). It includes English-, Spanish-, French-, and Dutch-speaking nations and territories of varying sizes. The region's average regional economic growth rate of about 2% over the past decade has been insufficient to generate adequate employment and reduce poverty, and individual countries are at varying stages of development. Some Caribbean countries, including Barbados, the Bahamas, Antigua, and Bermuda, are ranked high according to the U.N. Human Development Index, and most others, with the exception of Haiti, are ranked at a medium level. The region as a whole is undergoing a demographic transition-a process of population change consisting of a gradual evolution from high birth and death rates to low ones. Haiti with high birth and death rates is at the lowest stage of demographic transition, Jamaica, Bahamas and Barbados are at the highest. In some countries, including the Bahamas, the Dominican Republic, and Trinidad and Tobago, the urbanization process is far advanced (more than 60% of the population reside in urban areas); however, in other countries, including Haiti, large segments of the population still live in rural areas. Economic activity in the region varies and includes the export of petroleum in Trinidad and Tobago to heavy reliance on tourism and banana exports in the countries that are part of the Organization of Eastern Caribbean States (OECS).

Available data, presented in this chapter, suggest that the HIV/AIDS epidemic is spreading alarmingly in the Caribbean region. CARICOM estimates that more cases of HIV/AIDS were reported in the Caribbean between 1995 and 1998 than had been reported since the beginning of the epidemic in the early 1980s. Perhaps not surprisingly, given the region's heterogeneity, the epidemics in the Caribbean have different driving forces and transmission routes. Different countries have also varied in their responses to HIV/AIDS. As a result, the Caribbean region as a whole might be considered to have not a single HIV/AIDS epidemic, but a "mosaic" of epidemics (Confronting AIDS, 1998):

- *Haiti, Bahamas, Barbados, the Dominican Republic, and Guyana* have generalized epidemics, meaning that HIV has spread far beyond the original subpopulations with high-risk behavior,[5] and 5% or more of women attending prenatal clinics are infected. Better reporting system in Barbados and Bahamas are contributing to a better understanding of the magnitude of the epidemic.

- *Jamaica and Trinidad and Tobago* have concentrated HIV/AIDS epidemics, meaning that their national epidemics are still affecting primarily population groups practicing high-risk

---

5 High-risk behaviour is defined as engaging in unprotected (i.e., without a condom) sexual intercourse with many partners or sharing of unsterilized needles or other injecting equipment.

behaviors (among whom infection rates exceed 5%) but are set to spread more widely in the rest of the population.

- *Other countries in the Caribbean* either have insufficient information to be classified or have nascent epidemics, meaning HIV/AIDS prevalence is still low (less than 5%—even among people presumed to practice high-risk behavior).

Box 2-1. Overview of the Caribbean Region

Definitions of the territorial scope of the Caribbean vary. Probably the "social/cultural" definition of the "wider" Caribbean region is most relevant as it pertains to the HIV/AIDS epidemic within the region. The "wider" Caribbean region includes the following:

1. The sovereign-state members of the Caribbean Community (CARICOM), including both island-nations (Antigua and Barbuda, The Bahamas, Barbados, Dominica, Grenada, Haiti, Jamaica, Montserrat, Saint Kitts and Nevis, Saint Lucia, Saint Vincent and the Grenadines, and Trinidad and Tobago) and the mainland countries of Belize in Central America, and Guyana and Suriname in South America.

2. Spanish-speaking Cuba and the Dominican Republic.

3. The semiautonomous states of the Kingdom of the Netherlands (Aruba and the Netherlands Antilles islands of Bonaire, Curacao, Saint Marten, Statia, and Saba).

4. The British-dependent territories of Anguilla, Bermuda, British Virgin Islands, Cayman Islands, Montserrat, and the Turks and Caicos Islands.

5. The U.S. commonwealth of Puerto Rico and territory of the U.S. Virgin Islands.

6. The territories of the Republic of France consisting of French Guyana, St. Marten, Guadeloupe, and Martinique.

The Caribbean is a multiethnic region with many cultural differences. There are English-speaking countries (e.g., Trinidad and Tobago), Spanish-speaking countries (e.g., the Dominican Republic), French-speaking countries (e.g., Haiti), and Dutch-speaking countries (e.g., Suriname). The majority of the population is of African descent, but there are also people of European, Hispanic, and Asian ancestry (e.g., East Indians in Trinidad and Tobago and Guyana).

The mainland states of Belize, Guyana, and Suriname, which by virtue of language and cultural heritage, form part of the Caribbean region, are much larger in land mass than the island states of the Caribbean: Belize (29,963 km^2, population 215,000), Guyana (219,470 km^2, population 813,000), and Suriname (163,820 km^2, population 437,000). The island states of the Caribbean vary in size and population from Anguilla (91 km^2 and 8,000 inhabitants) to Jamaica 11,424 km^2 and a population of 2,447,000.

Historically, the Caribbean region has been strongly influenced by Europe and the United States. Many of the English-speaking Caribbean countries have modeled their educational system, the legal system and the political system on the United Kingdom. The countries of the English-speaking Caribbean have a combined population of around 6.7 million scattered over the vast Caribbean Sea, whose farthest points span about 3,500 kilometers between the coasts of Belize and Guyana. The Bahamas and the Dominican Republic are economically reliant on the United States. France and Holland also have strong links with some of the non-English speaking countries, for example Martinique and Curacao. Therefore, there has been much migration from these countries to the Caribbean. The Caribbean is also a major tourist destination, attracting visitors from many parts of the world. Similarly, over the past 40 years, for economic reasons, many Caribbean citizens have migrated primarily to the United States, Canada, and the United Kingdom. There is also much business travel within and outside the Caribbean.

The geographic, political, cultural, and linguistic diversity of the Caribbean region underscores both the complexities in understanding the patterns of HIV contagion and successful responses. Given that human movement throughout the Caribbean and between it and other geographic areas has been the basic foundation of this region's existence since its formative days of "triangular trade" of slavery and colonization, it is clear that an appropriate response to the HIV/AIDS epidemics must recognize the contributing factor of its geopolitical heterogeneity and the complete disregard by HIV of geopolitical boundaries.

Source: PAHO/WHO, 1997.

HIV/AIDS EPIDEMIOLOGICAL PATTERNS AND TRENDS IN THE CARIBBEAN

Official statistics on the prevalence and incidence of HIV/AIDS cases in the Caribbean are presented below. It is important to recognize, however, that these statistics reflect a high level of underreporting of such cases.

Prevalence of HIV/AIDS in the Caribbean[6]

In 1999, about 360,000 persons were reported to be living with HIV/AIDS in the Caribbean region (see Table 2-1). According to UNAIDS, underreporting varies between 30% and 75%. The prevalence of HIV among adults ages 15-49 in the Caribbean region is 2%. *The Caribbean region currently has the highest prevalence of HIV of any region of the world other than the AIDS-ravaged sub-Saharan Africa*, where the prevalence of HIV among adults ages 15 to 49 is reported to be 8.0%.

As discussed further below, the primary mode of HIV transmission among adults in the Caribbean region is sexual intercourse between men and women. For that reason, the percentage of women with HIV/AIDS is rising. As of 1999, about 35% of the adults affected with HIV in the Caribbean region were women.

Children under age 14 currently account for only a small part of the known HIV-infected population in the Caribbean region as a whole, but the pediatric share is growing. By late 1996, there had been 6,911 cases of HIV/AIDS diagnosed in children under age 14 in Latin America and the Caribbean. Most young children (about 75%) are infected by their HIV-infected mothers during pregnancy, delivery, or breast-feeding.

In some Caribbean countries, even though the numbers of children involved are still fairly small, pediatric cases account for a significant portion of the HIV/AIDS population. In fact, the data available as of 1995 showed that *certain countries in the Caribbean were among the countries with the highest percentage of pediatric HIV/AIDS cases in the Americas:* 18.2% of HIV/AIDS cases in the British Virgin Islands occurred among children, 8% in French Guyana, 8.8% in Antigua and Barbuda, 8.4% in the Bahamas, and 7.2% in Trinidad and Tobago (Health Conditions in the Americas, PAHO/WHO, 1998).

None of the Caribbean countries and territories have been spared from HIV/AIDS. It is important to note, however, that officially reported HIV/AIDS cases and estimates disguise a wide variation in prevalence among the countries in the region. *Some Caribbean countries have the highest prevalence of HIV/AIDS among adults in Latin American and the Caribbean* (see Table 2-2). The most affected countries are Haiti, the Bahamas, Barbados, and Guyana, with an HIV prevalence rate among adults that ranges between about 2% and 5%. *Haiti, with an HIV prevalence rate of 5.17%, is the most affected country in the world outside of sub-Saharan Africa.* Cuba, on the other hand, has one of the lowest rates in the Americas (.02%). In terms of numbers of HIV/AIDS cases in the Caribbean, two countries stand out. *Haiti and the Dominican Republic, taken together, account for 85% of the total number of cases in the Caribbean.*

---

6 Prevalence is a commonly used epidemiological term that refers to the percentage of people suffering from an illness or condition at a given time. Prevalence rates are typically expressed as a percentage of the total population. Thus, the prevalence of HIV is defined as the percentage of the total population that is infected with HIV, including both HIV-positive individuals who have not yet developed AIDS and individuals whose HIV infection has developed into AIDS. From a public health point of view, HIV prevalence is important because it provides a measure of the population's general risk of contracting AIDS. The higher the prevalence of HIV, the higher the risk of contracting AIDS.

Table 2-1. World HIV/AIDS Statistics by Region, December 1999

Region	Epidemic started	Adults & children living with HIV/AIDS	Adults & children newly infected with HIV	Adult prevalence rate (*)	Percent of HIV-positive adults who are women	Main mode(s) of transmission (#) for adults living with HIV/AIDS
Sub-Saharan Africa	Late '70s	23.3 million	3.8 million	8.0%	55%	Hetero
North Africa & Middle East	Late '80s	220,000	19,000	0.13%	20%	IDU, Hetero
South & South-East Asia	Late '80s	6 million	1.3 million	0.69%	30%	Hetero
East Asia & Pacific	Late '80s	530,000	120,000	0.068%	15%	IDU, Hetero MSM
Latin America	Late '70s	1.3 million	150,000	0.57%	20%	MSM, IDU, Hetero
Caribbean	Late '70s Early '80s	360,000	57,000	1.96%	35%	Hetero, MSM
Eastern Europe & Central Asia	Early '90s	360,000	95,000	0.14%	20%	IDU, MSM
Western Europe	Late '70s early '80s	520,000	30,000	0.25%	20%	MSM, IDU
North America	Late '70s Early '80s	920,000	44,000	0.56%	20%	MSM, IDU, Hetero
Australia & New Zealand	Late '70s Early '80s	12,000	500	0.1%	10%	MSM, IDU
TOTAL		33.6 million	5.6 million	1.1%	46%	

* The percentage of adults ages 15 to 49 living with HIV/AIDS in 1999, based on 1998 population numbers.
KEY: Hetero (heterosexual transmission of HIV); MSM (sexual transmission of HIV among men who have sex with men); IDU (transmission of HIV through injecting drug use).
Source: UNAIDS, 1999.

According to UNAIDS, which has estimated the number of HIV/AIDS cases taking into account such underreporting, several factors contribute to an underestimation of the size and scope of the HIV/AIDS problem in the Caribbean:

- A lack of a standardized case definition in the region as a whole, which makes consistent diagnosis and uniform reporting difficult.

- Few and outdated sentinel surveillance studies to determine HIV seroprevalence[7] over time.

- A lack of national policies in the Caribbean regarding testing and reporting of HIV.

- Limited or no access to voluntary, confidential HIV counseling and testing

- Underreporting, late reporting, or no reporting of cases.

---

7 Seroprevalence: the prevalence of an infection in a given population as detected in blood serum.

- Residents' fear of being tested for HIV, given that a positive test result may lead to marginalization or exclusion from society and the workplace.

- Residents' traveling abroad to be tested because of concerns about confidentiality

Adjusting official statistics to account for underreporting, UNAIDS has estimated that more than 500,000 people in the Caribbean region (as opposed to the 360,000 officially reported) may currently be infected with HIV.

Incidence of AIDS in the Caribbean[8]

The first AIDS case in the Caribbean is traced back to the 1970s. By the end of 1985, all of the Caribbean countries had reported at least one AIDS case. Since then, the reported number of new AIDS cases per million population has been climbing every year. Currently, *the Caribbean region has the highest incidence of reported AIDS cases in the Americas, and the trend is not encouraging* (see Figure 2-1).

AIDS incidence rates have been increasing significantly in the English-speaking Caribbean, which together constitutes the majority of the member countries of CARICOM. In the English-speaking Caribbean countries, the AIDS incidence rate rose from 142.3 AIDS cases per million in 1991 to 246.2 per million in 1996. In the Latin Caribbean countries, although Cuba remains with a low AIDS incidence rate, data from Haiti and the Dominican Republic show a similar upward trend. If Puerto Rico is included in the Latin Caribbean figures, the observed trend becomes more pronounced.

Table 2.2. HIV/AIDS Prevalence Rates Among Adults (Ages 15-49) in Countries in Latin America and the Caribbean, December 1997

Rank	Country	HIV/AIDS Prevalence Rate (%)
1	Haiti	5.17
2	Bahamas	3.77
3	Barbados	2.89
4	Guyana	2.13
5	Belize	1.89
	Dominican Republic	1.89
6	Honduras	1.46
7	Suriname	1.17
8	Jamaica	0.99
9	Trinidad & Tobago	0.94
10	Argentina	0.69
	Venezuela	0.69
11	Brazil	0.63
12	Panama	0.61
13	El Salvador	0.58
14	Peru	0.56
15	Costa Rica	0.55
16	Guatemala	0.52
17	Colombia	0.36
18	Mexico	0.35
19	Uruguay	0.33
20	Ecuador	0.28
21	Chile	0.20
22	Nicaragua	0.19
23	Paragua	0.13
24	Bolivia	0.07
25	Cuba	0.02

Note: Adult rates (%) are derived from the number of adults (15-49 years) living with HIV/AIDS at the end of 1997 divided by the 1997 adult population.

Source: UNAIDS, Report on the Global HIV/AIDS Epidemic, June 1998, PAHO/WHO, 2000

---

8 Incidence, in contrast to prevalence, is defined as the number of *new* cases of a disease occurring in the population during a specified period of time. Thus, the incidence of AIDS is often presented as the number of new cases of AIDS diagnosed during a given year per million population. Many years typically lapse between the time an individual is infected with HIV and the time he or she develops full-blown AIDS. For that reason, AIDS incidence rates reflect rates of HIV infection from years before. Absent widespread screening for HIV, most cases of HIV/AIDS are only detected when individuals develop and begin to exhibit symptoms of AIDS. For this reason, statistics on the incidence of AIDS cases may be thought of as only the "tip of the iceberg," because many people who are infected with HIV in the population have not yet developed visible signs of AIDS.

The growing importance of the HIV/AIDS epidemic in most countries of the Caribbean can be better appreciated if one compares the incidence figures in these countries with the steady downward trend in AIDS incidence rates that has been observed in North America (Canada and the United States) since 1992—from 280.9 AIDS cases per million in 1992 to 126.9 per million in 1996, in large part due to improved access to medical care.

Official AIDS incidence rates among the Caribbean Epidemiology Center (CAREC) member countries[9] have steadily increased since the 1980s (see Figure 2-2). CAREC reports that the cumulative number of officially reported AIDS cases in CAREC countries increased from 9,978 at the end of 1996 to 14,380 in 1998. In terms of cumulative AIDS cases per 100,000 population in CAREC countries as of 1996, the country with the highest number was the Bahamas, with 146.6 AIDS cases per 100,000 population; next highest were Bermuda (66.0), Barbados (50.3), Trinidad and Tobago (33.4), and Jamaica (22.3).

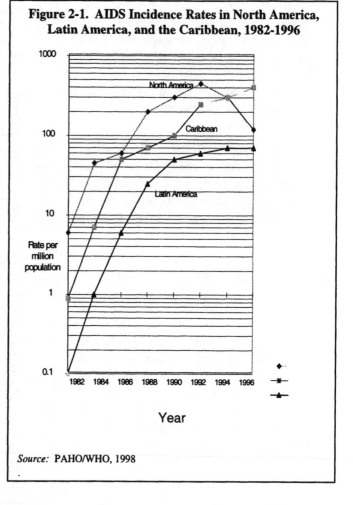

Figure 2-1. AIDS Incidence Rates in North America, Latin America, and the Caribbean, 1982-1996

Source: PAHO/WHO, 1998

The HIV/AIDS epidemic has been moving into younger and younger population groups. About 83% of AIDS cases are diagnosed in people between the ages of 15 and 54, and almost half of these cases are diagnosed in people ages 25 to 34. These figures suggest, given an estimated average incubation period of eight to 10 years from HIV infection to the development of AIDS, that about half of new HIV infections are occurring among young people ages 15 to 24. The affected age group are those forming the labor force. Among men, the majority of AIDS cases are in the 30-34 and 25-29 age cohort; among women, the majority of cases are in the 25-29 year-old age bracket, followed by the 30-34 year age group (PAHO/WHO, 1998).

---

9 PAHO/WHO reporting of HIV/AIDS statistics for the Caribbean region is usually broken down into two categories: *CAREC countries* (Anguilla, Antigua and Barbuda, Bahamas, Barbados, Bermuda, Belize, British Virgin Islands, Cayman Islands, Dominica, Grenada, Guyana, Jamaica, Montserrat, St. Kitts and Nevis, St. Lucia, St. Vincent and the Grenadines, Trinidad and Tobago, Turks and Caicos Islands, and Suriname); and the *Latin Caribbean group* (Cuba, Dominican Republic, and Haiti).

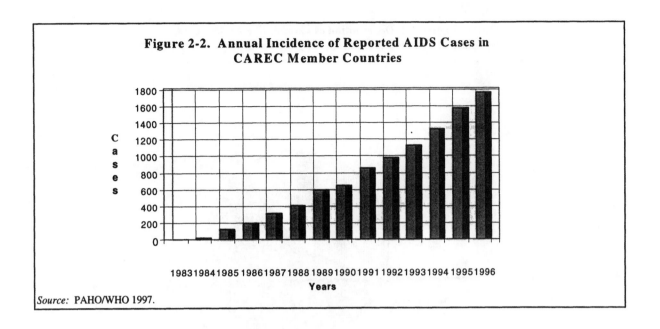

Figure 2-2. Annual Incidence of Reported AIDS Cases in CAREC Member Countries

Source: PAHO/WHO 1997.

MODES OF HIV TRANSMISSION IN THE CARIBBEAN

In Latin America and the Caribbean, *unprotected sexual contact is the main transmission mechanism for HIV/AIDS*. More than half of all the AIDS cases that have occurred in the Caribbean region to date were the result of reported unprotected sexual intercourse between men and women. In the English-speaking Caribbean, heterosexual contact accounts about 60% of reported AIDS cases (see Figure 2-3), while in the Latin Caribbean it represents about 50% of the reported AIDS cases. The following factors have a large influence on the rate of sexual transmission of HIV and other STDs (Confronting AIDS, 1998):

- The longer a person remains infectious.

- The more frequent a person has sexual contacts.

- The more new sexual partners contacted.

Other modes of HIV transmission in the Caribbean region, as discussed further below, are homosexual/bisexual unprotected sexual relations; the use of contaminated needles by intravenous drug users; blood-borne transmission; and, increasingly, mother-to-child transmission. The percentage of AIDS cases due to mother-to-child transmission of HIV in the Caribbean is now the highest in the Americas.

Heterosexual Transmission of HIV

Sex between men and women has quickly outpaced HIV transmission by other means. Heterosexual transmission has been the main route of HIV transmission since 1986, facilitated by a number of factors, which are discussed in Chapter III. Women are more vulnerable to HIV than men for biological reasons (i.e., their anatomy makes them more vulnerable than men), as well as for social and cultural norms (i.e., machismo; male-female power relations whereby many women have little or no power to negotiate safer sex practices with their male partners). About 35% of the adults living with HIV/AIDS in the Caribbean region are women.

**Figure 2-3. Distribution of Cumulative AIDS Cases,
by Mode of Transmission, in the English-Speaking Caribbean, 1998**

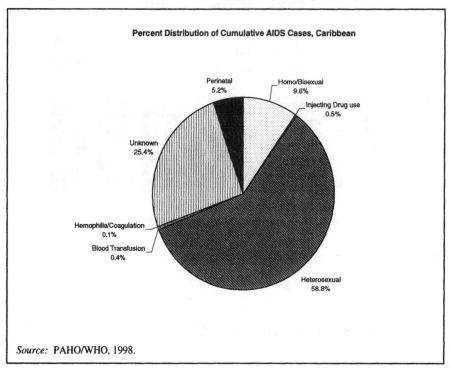

Percent Distribution of Cumulative AIDS Cases, Caribbean

Perinatal 5.2%

Homo/Bisexual 9.6%

Injecting Drug use 0.5%

Unknown 25.4%

Hemophilia/Coagulation 0.1%

Blood Transfusion 0.4%

Heterosexual 58.8%

Source: PAHO/WHO, 1998.

Currently, *the Caribbean region has one of the highest rates of new AIDS cases among women in the Americas.* The male-to-female ratio for reported HIV infections cases has been declining in both the Caribbean and Latin America in the 1990s. In the early part of the decade, the ratios were 4.9:1 in Latin America and 2:1 in the Caribbean, whereas in 1996, they were 3.2:1 and 1.7:1, respectively. According to PAHO/WHO, the declining male-to-female ratio of HIV infections reflects the growing "feminization" of the HIV/AIDS epidemic in these regions.

In Haiti, the ratio of male-to-female HIV infections is almost 1:1 (i.e., almost evenly split between genders), and the HIV/AIDS epidemic has spread broadly to 8% of pregnant women—as a result, there is significant mother-to-child transmission of HIV in that country. Similarly, in Guyana, nearly 7% of women attending prenatal clinics were infected with HIV as of 1992. In the Dominican Republic, more than 70% of AIDS cases are attributed to heterosexual transmission; there, the male-to-female ratio of cases now stands at 2:1 and is declining. The prevalence of HIV among pregnant women is 2.8% nationwide in that country, and in some areas it has reached 8%. The male-to-female ratio of HIV infections in other countries, including Dominica, Barbados, Antigua, and Trinidad and Tobago, ranges between 3.6:1 and 2.4:1.

Men-Who-Have-Sex-with-Men Transmission of HIV

Reported homosexual and bisexual transmission of HIV is relatively low in the Caribbean, accounting for about 10% of AIDS cases, but MSM transmission is nonetheless considered an important mode of HIV transmission. Given discrimination against homosexuals and bisexuals in the Caribbean it is quite likely that the reported data underestimate the true percentage of AIDS cases attributable to MSM transmission of HIV.

According to CAREC, approximately 20% of AIDS cases among men in the English-speaking Caribbean are reported to be due to sexual contact with other men, whereas 22% of cases of cases among men are reported as "mode of transmission: unknown." Of the 22%, it is assumed that most are probably through male-to-male sex.

Injecting-Drug-Use Transmission of HIV

In most Caribbean countries, the transmission of HIV by injecting drug use is reported to be minimal, ranging from 0% to 2% of AIDS cases. Bermuda is the exception, where injecting-drug-use transmission represents 43% of total reported AIDS cases. Puerto Rico, reflected in United States statistics, represents another Caribbean community heavily affected by injecting drug use. Crack-cocaine drug use has been shown to be associated with higher risk of HIV infection in the Bahamas, Trinidad and Tobago, and Jamaica. Among crack-cocaine users, HIV seroprevalence can be as high as 42% in Bahamas and Trinidad and Tobago (CAREC, 1999).

Mother-to-Child and Blood-Borne Transmission of HIV

The percentage of AIDS cases where children were infected by HIV-positive mothers is higher in the Caribbean region than in any other part of the Americas. Recent estimates indicate that following the increase in the number of AIDS cases among women, mother-to-child or vertical transmission now accounts for 6% of all reported AIDS cases in CAREC countries. Mother-to-child transmission is more likely to happen depending on the stage of the disease that the woman is in, the viral load and procedures carried out during birth. The transmission of HIV through blood or blood products account for less than 3% of AIDS cases in the Caribbean.

POPULATIONS AT HIGH RISK OF HIV INFECTION IN THE CARIBBEAN

Populations at high-risk are young people who engage in unprotected sexual intercourse, and men who engage in sexual intercourse with other men. The newborns of HIV-infected women are another group at high risk.

Many countries in the Caribbean have set up surveillance systems to track the spread of HIV through their populations. The specific type of surveillance necessary follows the general pattern of infection in a given country. Sentinel surveillance of population groups in the Caribbean have primarily included commercial sex workers, people attending STD clinics, and pregnant women. These groups are discussed below.

Commercial Sex Workers

Commercial sex workers are defined as women or men who provide sex for material gain. In the Caribbean, as noted by CARICOM (2000), commercial sex work is widespread and increasing throughout the countries. It is linked to tourism and to other economic endeavors such as mining, migrant farming and informal sector hawking. Economic hardship is the primary motivating factor for sex work.

Prevalence among sex workers has been rising over the course of the epidemic. The problem is aggravated by the absence of any regulation in the sex trade industry and the marginalized status of the trade, implying that social and health services are rarely responsive to the particular needs of commercial sex workers (CARICOM, 2000). In Haiti, 42% to 53% of this population group in the largest urban areas is infected; in the Dominican Republic, the figures varied between 5% and 6% in 1994-95 (PAHO/WHO, 1998). The epidemic has also infected significant numbers of commercial sex workers in Guyana, Jamaica, and Trinidad and Tobago. In Guyana, a survey of commercial sex workers found a seroprevalence of 25% in 1993. In Jamaica, HIV prevalence among commercial sex workers in Kingston was 11% in 1995, but were higher in Montego Bay at 22%. Surveys of commercial sex workers in Trinidad and Tobago have also found high rates of HIV infection (European Union, 1998).

Attendees of Clinics for Treating STDs

STDs are common in the Caribbean (PAHO/WHO, 1996). Studies in both industrial and developing countries indicate that people with current or past STDs are two to nine times more likely to be infected with HIV (Confronting AIDS, 1998). HIV infection rates are high among STD clinic attendees in several Caribbean countries, reflecting the close interaction between HIV/AIDS infection and STDs. In Jamaica, HIV prevalence among STD clinic attendees rose from 0.25% in 1986 to 3.1% in 1990 and 6.3% in 1997. Among STD clinic "repeaters," HIV prevalence was higher; 10% in 1990 and 9.3% in 1993. In Guyana, HIV prevalence among STD clinic attendees was as high as 13.1% in 1992 and 6.6% among women and 21.0% among men in 1995. In Trinidad and Tobago and the Bahamas, HIV prevalence among STD clinic attendees peaked at 13.6% in 1991/92 and declined to 6-7% in 1995/96. Among Haitian migrant workers living in the bateyes, or sugarcane plantations, of the Dominican Republic in 1995, there was high prevalence of STDs, including 5.7% for HIV (PAHO/WHO, 1998).

Pregnant Women

HIV prevalence among pregnant women has been monitored in several countries through sentinel surveillance. CAREC (1999) estimated that in 1997 there was an HIV prevalence rate of 1-2% among pregnant women in the Caribbean.

Haiti has the highest prevalence of HIV among women receiving prenatal care services in the Latin Caribbean (ranging from 8% to 9% between 1986 and 1993 in urban areas and from 3% to 4% in rural areas between 1986 and 1990). In the Dominican Republic the figures ranged from 1% in 1991 to 4%-8% in 1998. In Cuba there is no sign of infection among this population (PAHO/WHO, 1998).

In the English-speaking Caribbean, the prevalence of HIV infection among women receiving prenatal care services is less than 1% in the Bahamas, Grenada, the Cayman Islands, Saint Vincent and the Grenadines, Suriname, and Trinidad and Tobago (PAHO/WHO, 1998). In Jamaica, HIV seroprevalence among prenatal clinic attendees increased from 1.4 per 1,000 in 1989 to 9.5 in 1997. In Barbados, HIV seroprevalence varied between 8 and 12 per 1,000 between 1992 and 1996. In Guyana, a survey of pregnant women in 1992 found an HIV infection prevalence of 7%. In the Bahamas, country-wide HIV screening of pregnant women was introduced on a voluntary basis. HIV prevalence among pregnant women was highest in 1993 at 4.8% and declined to 4.2% in 1994 and 3.6% in 1995.

MORTALITY DUE TO AIDS IN THE CARIBBEAN

During the last two decades, there were 6,566 AIDS deaths reported in the region, representing 1.4% of total AIDS deaths in the Americas (PAHO/WHO, 1998). The actual number of deaths due to AIDS in the Caribbean is probably higher than the officially reported number (given the probability of underreporting or inaccurate diagnosis of cause of death).

The AIDS case fatality rate[10] in the Caribbean region as a whole is high, 63% in 1996. *In the English-speaking Caribbean, AIDS is now the largest cause of death among young men between the ages of 15 and 44.* Recent research in the Dominican Republic shows that AIDS is the most common cause of death among women in their reproductive ages in the geographic area studied, the National District of Santo Domingo, which encompasses about 30% of the country's population. About 12% of all deaths among the women of childbearing age in that region were found to be caused by AIDS; the next most common cause of death was violence. Unfortunately, mortality from AIDS disproportionately affects young women: 56% of all deaths due to AIDS occur in individuals between 20 and 34 years of age (Cáceres Uraña, 1998).

One of the most devastating impacts of deaths from HIV/AIDS is on the children of parents who are victims of the disease. HIV/AIDS most frequently strikes adults who are often raising children and are at the prime of their working lives. By the end of 1999, *the cumulative number of Caribbean children estimated to have been orphaned by HIV/AIDS at age 14 or younger stood at 83,000* (UNAIDS, 1999). Experience in other regions of the world has demonstrated that deaths and illness due to AIDS among adults has a profoundly negative impact on the welfare of children in the affected households. Frequently, poor health and premature death of adults lead to income and expenditures changes that can have adverse effects on child nutrition and schooling (Confronting AIDS, 1998; Dasgupta et al. 1999). Some families can no longer afford school costs or the children are needed to help out at home. Children's education may also suffer as a result, reducing literacy rates in communities. This would be particularly onerous for poor families given the already stratified educational system in the Caribbean that is reflected in higher attrition of poor students at all grade levels that becomes deeper and wider at each successive level, and in a skewed distribution of resources to the detriment of schools in poorer communities (Caribbean Education Sector Strategy 2020, World Bank, 2000).

According to UNAIDS (2000), AIDS case fatality rates have remained at a constant high in the Caribbean due to several factors:

- Late diagnosis of HIV infection and related conditions.

- Lack of policies, skills, and resources in preventing mother-to-child HIV transmission in many countries.

- Lack of accessibility to antiretroviral (ARV) drugs use to treat HIV-positive individuals in countries such as the United States.

- Lack of access to basic medicines to combat opportunistic infections.

- Lack or denial of services to HIV/AIDS patients in some countries.

In some countries of the Caribbean, HIV/AIDS has pushed back or is starting to reverse the gains in life expectancy achieved in previous decades as the result of progress in the fight against communicable diseases. In Haiti and Guyana, life expectancy is estimated to be 5.7 and 5.2 years less, respectively, than it would have been without AIDS (UNAIDS, 2000). *What is ominous for the Caribbean region, however, is that even if all HIV transmission could be halted today, the impact of the illness and deaths of the people already infected will be felt over the next two decades.*

---

10 The case fatality rate is the number of deaths from a disease during a defined period of time expressed as a percentage of the total number of people with the disease.

SOCIOECONOMIC IMPACTS OF AIDS IN THE CARIBBEAN

HIV has a long latency period, so some of the social and economic consequences of the HIV/AIDS epidemic may not be felt immediately. Eventually, however, if the prevalence of HIV continues to increase in the Caribbean as it has been, per capita economic growth may begin to decline. Increased expenditures for treatment of AIDS and AIDS-related diseases from government budgets and household savings will reduce the capital for more productive investments.

Preliminary efforts have been made to project the expected macroeconomic impact of HIV/AIDS within Caribbean countries by the years 2005 and 2020. A macroeconomic impact study of Jamaica and Trinidad and Tobago revealed contractions in major variables, such as the Gross Domestic Product (declines of 6.4 and 4.2 percent, respectively). The level of investment was also severely affected as incomes had to be redirected from the production of goods and services to finance HIV- related expenditures. These HIV-related illness expenditures rose by 25.3% in Trinidad and Tobago and 35.4% in Jamaica. Even using low case scenario data, impacts upon several key industries were evidenced, the service sector categories were more greatly affected than employment in agriculture or manufacturing (Camara at al, 1997).

The emergence of AIDS as a major health problem places a tremendous burden on the health care systems of the Caribbean countries. Assessments conducted by the University of the West Indies (UNAIDS, 1998) suggest that HIV/AIDS may have important fiscal consequences in the Caribbean, as national health budgets are increasingly taxed by the costs of care for HIV-infected people (e.g., the biggest burden to the health care system is that for managing the opportunistic infections, such as tuberculosis, chronic and severe diarrhea, and other complications, that all put a burden on the bed capacity of hospitals and outpatient departments). The case management of HIV or AIDS through the prophylactic administration of an antiretroviral drug like zidovudine (AZT), that costs more than US$3,000 per year, would represent more than three times the national per capita income in many Caribbean countries. AIDS drains scarce skills and resources needed for addressing other health priorities such as childhood diseases or malaria.

HIV/AIDS has considerable potential to cause a negative impact on economic sectors such as agriculture, tourism, mining, lumber, finance, and trade as a result of lost productivity of economically active adults with HIV/AIDS and premature death. The shock of AIDS to the labor markets is one mechanism through which AIDS might adversely affect economic growth in the Caribbean. At present, the affected age group (83% of AIDS cases in the Caribbean are in the age group 15-54 years) are those forming the labor force. A survey of people living with HIV/AIDS in the Caribbean indicate that most of them were already unemployed due in some cases to workplace attitudes (Wint, 2000).

As noted in a United Nations Security Council meeting convened in early January 2000, the first time to take up a health issue, HIV/AIDS has grown beyond a health epidemic to become a threat to global security and stability. In a similar fashion, the United States government in April 2000 formally designated the disease as a threat to U.S. national security because the epidemic could undo decades of development work in the world. These concerns are highly relevant for the Caribbean because its HIV/AIDS epidemic could create significant externalities beyond the region (e.g., according to recent health data, the fastest growing epidemic within Canada is amongst Canadians from the Caribbean, mainly Haitian in Montreal; the second highest urban HIV seroprevalence in the United States is found in San Juan, Puerto Rico). The high-profile international attention to this issue implies that Caribbean governments cannot deny or ignore it anymore.

THE TASK AHEAD

The forces driving the HIV/AIDS epidemic and the implications of the epidemic in the Caribbean are inextricably linked to the region's economic, social, and cultural dynamics. Caribbean AIDS experts have put forth a number of specific challenges to addressing the problem of HIV/AIDS in the region, including the following:

- A large discrepancy between cultural, moral, and religious taboos and actual sexual practices in Caribbean countries.

- A lack of information and HIV/AIDS prevention programs targeted to groups most at risk (e.g., young people, commercial sex workers, men who have sex with men, migrants).

- Low approval rate of condom use among men and women, coupled with the church opposition to condom use.

- Stigmatization of and discrimination against persons living with HIV/AIDS, which contribute to HIV transmission by discouraging the use of HIV testing and other services.

- Low use of health care facilities for managing HIV/AIDS and other STDs, both in the public and the private sectors, due in part to concerns about confidentiality and the lack of access to effective HIV/AIDS therapies.

- The lack of antiretroviral drugs for most HIV-infected people and people with AIDS in the Caribbean.

As discussed in the next chapter, Caribbean governments and their partners have taken several actions to combat the HIV/AIDS epidemic, but these actions have not yet turned the epidemic around. It is important for Caribbean governments, with the support of their development partners, to act decisively now before the epidemic reaches the levels it has in sub-Saharan Africa. A key challenge will be putting more effective HIV/AID prevention programs into place. As governments operate with resource constraints and fixed budgets, the call for greater actions in health protection and promotion and disease prevention cannot ignore their cost and how these services will be paid for. The World Bank's *1993 World Development Report* (World Bank, 1993) recommends that developing countries use an approach for setting priorities that involves comparing the likely costs and impacts of different preventive and curative interventions. This approach is an important resource allocation tool because cost-effective interventions such as greater use of condoms, cost as little as U\$8 per infection averted, whereas the treatment of opportunistic infections associated with AIDS and anti-HIV treatment, which does not cure AIDS, costs thousands of dollars per year per patient.

> " *Those who cannot remember the past are condemned to repeat it.* "

> *George Santayana*
> *Poet and Philosopher*

III INTENSIFYING ACTION AGAINST HIV/AIDS: KEY CHALLENGES FOR CARIBBEAN COUNTRIES

HOW HAVE CARIBBEAN COUNTRIES RESPONDED TO THE HIV/AIDS EPIDEMIC?

Starting from the early days of the HIV/AIDS epidemic, Caribbean countries and territories established National AIDS Programs and developed short- and medium-term plans for responding to the epidemic. Caribbean governments—in partnership with regional and international agencies, including those in the United Nations System (UNAIDS), CAREC, bilateral cooperation agencies, and national and international nongovernmental organizations (NGOs)—have sought to address the various aspects of the epidemic in the region. The actions taken with support of these partners have included advocacy and social mobilization, regional and national policy development, the establishment of HIV prevention and drug-control activities and programs, the development of mass media campaigns, and prevention program and services for young people.

As a result, throughout the Caribbean region, there are country- level successes to identify pertaining to HIV/ AIDS responses. The safety of blood supply in the vast majority of the region is due to both early intervention as well as pre-existing relative strengths in the areas of public health laboratory work. For the smaller island-states of the eastern Caribbean in particular, Caribbean Epidemiology Center (CAREC)'s assistance has been helpful. Jamaica has confronted STDs vigorously over the years. The Dominican Republic has elevated its national HIV/IDS program to the level of the president's office in order to demonstrate the serious commitment and the multisectoral responsibility. Since 1986, Cuba has established an effective strategy for addressing HIV/AIDS, including conducting studies of the groups at highest risk, carrying out epidemiological investigation of 100% of cases, performing analyses of hospital admission and outpatient care records, and implementing a comprehensive program of health education for the general population. For many years, the Dutch Caribbean has had outreach programs for commercial sex workers that includes voluntary counseling and testing, STD control, condom distribution and information in the several languages of these migratory CSWs. Barbados has been recognized for its comprehensive, school-based HIV/AIDS education efforts in secondary schools. Through Martinique and Dominica, the French government not only supplies antiretroviral treatment for its Caribbean citizens, but also provides support for nationals of independent Dominica.

Yet, despite these individual components of success, what is needed in most of the Caribbean countries is a comprehensive, multisectoral national response that engages government, civil society, and international donors, as well as scaled up efforts to serve entire national populations, as the HIV/AIDS epidemic continues unabated in the region. Health services in Caribbean countries are struggling to respond to the growing population of individuals, including women and children, with HIV/AIDS who require care, support, and treatment. The general level of public understanding of how to prevent HIV/AIDS throughout the Caribbean is low, as it is in many parts of the world. The institutional capacity and the financial resources available to governments needed to contain transmission and treat people living with HIV/AIDS are inadequate. A sense of individual and collective mission and leadership needs to be fostered.

Fortunately, there is still an opportunity in the Caribbean to prevent HIV/AIDS rates from escalating to the alarming levels found in many sub-Saharan African countries. Concerted action by Caribbean governments and Caribbean regional agencies, in partnership with the private sector and NGOs and with the assistance of the international community, can make a difference. A further investment in the control of HIV *now* will mitigate the adverse impact of AIDS on the people and economics of the Caribbean region in the years that lie ahead.

STOPPING THE SPREAD OF HIV/AIDS—WHAT WORKS?

There is a broad consensus about what steps must be taken in order to combat the spread of HIV/AIDS. Worldwide, successful HIV/AIDS responses have several elements in common (see Box 3-1).

Box 3-1. Stopping the Spread of HIV/AIDS—What Works?

Successful programs against the HIV/AIDS epidemic to date have had several key features:

- *Government commitment* at the highest level and multiple partnerships at all levels with civil society and the private sector

- *Cooperation and collaboration among many different groups and sectors*: those who are most affected by the epidemic, religious and community leaders, (NGOs, researchers and health professionals, and the private sector

- *Decentralised and participatory approaches* that bring prevention and care programs to a truly national scale

- *A forward-looking, comprehensive and multisectoral response* that addresses the socioeconomic determinants that make people vulnerable to infection, and targets prevention interventions, care, treatment, and support

- *Community participation*—including people living with HIV/AIDS, NGOs, civil society, and the private sector—in government policymaking, design and implementation of programs.

Source: CARICOM/Caribbean Task Force on HIV/AIDS, 2000.

In order to be successful, HIV/AIDS prevention campaigns in Caribbean countries must be concentrated at three basic levels: (1) preventing sexual transmission of HIV in young people and adults, (2) preventing mother-to-child transmission of HIV, and (3) preventing blood-borne transmission of HIV (e.g., contaminated blood supplies, use of contaminated needles or other instruments).

Preventing the Sexual Transmission of HIV

As noted in Chapter II, unprotected sexual contact with a person infected with HIV is the primary mechanism by which HIV is transmitted in the Caribbean region, and the majority of cases are reported transmitted through heterosexual contact. Homosexual transmission of HIV also occurs among men having sex with men in the region. In most Caribbean countries, most people are aware of AIDS, but many people still lack detailed knowledge about modes of HIV transmission and do not know how to protect themselves from the disease. It is especially important to prevent the sexual transmission of HIV among young people, who tend to initiate sexual activity at an early age in the Caribbean.

Important considerations in developing approaches to prevent the sexual transmission of HIV/AIDS in Caribbean countries include the following:

- *Machismo and other cultural factors.* To prove their *machismo*, many men in Caribbean countries (and elsewhere in the world) engage in high-risk behaviors such as having early and frequent sex with multiple women. Such behaviors amplify both their own vulnerability and their partners' vulnerability to HIV infection. Because "macho" men are expected to know about sex, they are discouraged by social and cultural norms from obtaining access to information and services for safer sex. Since women are often economically and emotionally dependent on their male partner and are expected to defer to male demands and decisionmaking even when they know their partner may be infected through outside relationships. The 1998 Caribbean Adolescent Health Survey conducted by PAHO found considerable violence against and sexual abuse of young women. Sexual violence in childhood is the greatest determinant of high-risk sexual activity during adolescence. In Haiti, about 300,000 youngsters are working as domestic servants, many of them in situations where they are physically and sexually abused. Finally, the tension between *machismo* and homosexuality complicates the task of informing men who engage in sex with other men about HIV prevention. It is worth mentioning that in most Caribbean countries, homosexuality and commercial sex work are criminal offences. This stigmatizes certain high risk groups and behaviours and further drives the problem underground.

- *Economic and political conditions.* Some men and women, and even children, in the Caribbean are forced by economic or political conditions to leave their families to find work or to become commercial sex workers in order to survive. Migrant workers, such as those living in single-sex dormitories far away from their families, frequently turn to commercial sex workers for sex. They then go home and infect their spouses or partners with STDs such as syphilis and/or HIV. Commercial sex workers, particularly women, in the Caribbean often move from one city or island to another, carrying HIV infection as they go. In the Dominican Republic, widespread commercial sex is one of the key factors behind the AIDS epidemic. In some countries, thousands of impoverished children are living on the streets, and these children often turn to sex to survive or are subjected to rape. In Haiti, for example, there are an estimated 5,000 Haitian children living on the streets. These children are at high risk for contracting STDs and HIV.

- *Early initiation of sexual activity among young people.* Many young people in the Caribbean initiate sexual activity—generally unprotected—at a young age, making them extremely vulnerable to HIV and other STDs. The 1998 Caribbean Adolescent Health Survey conducted by PAHO in 100 schools in Antigua, Dominican Republic, Grenada and Jamaica and with out-of-school youth showed that, among those who reported being sexually active, more than 40% said their sexual debut had started before age 10 and another 20% said it had started at age 11 or 12. In some places, young people in rural areas become sexually active earlier than city-dwellers—in the Dominican Republic, 67.7% as against 47.1%.

- *Tourism.* The Caribbean is the most tourism dependent region in the world. Travel and tourism are expected to generate US$32 billion dollars of economic activity in 1998, and contribute 25% of GDP. Each year for the past several years, more than 30 million people— tourists and cruise passengers—have visited one or more of the thirty-two countries that are members of the Caribbean Tourism Organization (CTO) for vacation and recreation. The persistent trend of the time has been an average increase of 5.8% per annum. (Marshall, 1998). Among the tourists are "sex tourists," who engage in unsafe sex practices with fellow tourists and local residents (e.g., female commercial sex workers, "beach boys," children). Such tourism has been more often identified in Spanish and Dutch Caribbean destinations, but also in Haiti and the English-speaking Caribbean countries. The discussion of links between HIV transmission and tourism have often spawned concerns in tourism- based economies worldwide that any correlation between the two could cause financial ruin. However, in countries that have confronted this issue directly, such as Thailand, they have been able to avert any such economic impact and also curb the spread of HIV (Marshall, 1998).

- *Drug use.* Drug use is seen in many countries in the Caribbean and can start very early—for example, among children living or working on the streets. Intravenous drug users in the Caribbean run a high risk of becoming infected with HIV by sharing needles used to inject drugs. Non-injection drug use, including alcohol, crack-cocaine and marijuana, have been connected with HIV transmission due to their impacts upon sexual libido, decision-making and action. Given the prevalence of these and similarly-effecting drugs within the Caribbean, this must be a critical concern for future prevention efforts.

Programs to prevent sexual transmission of HIV among children and young people

Reaching young people is a key element in the prevention of the AIDS epidemic in the Caribbean since youth in the Caribbean are at high risk of HIV. It is also important to stress that a large percentage of the Caribbean population is comprised of young people. In Haiti, for instance, over half of the population is under 20 years of age and birthrates are increasing rapidly.

Young people between the ages of 10 and 25 represent half of the people who become infected with HIV. For that reason, young people need to have the understanding, motivation, skills, tools, and freedom to adopt behaviors that protect them from HIV infection. As noted earlier, children in Caribbean countries typically initiate sexual activity at a young age. Generally, youngsters who begin having sex at an early age (whether consensual or forced) do not use condoms and are therefore vulnerable not only to unwanted pregnancy and STDs such as syphilis, but also infection with HIV.

In view of the early onset of sexual intercourse among young people in the Caribbean, it is essential that parents and schools begin discussions with their children about AIDS and how to protect themselves when children are at a young age. The Health and Family Life Education (HFLE), which has been endorsed by CARICOM and a variety of other partners, is an example of a program based on the notion that promoting behavioral change among young people requires empowering students in a variety of realms (see Box 3-2).

Schools are a prime setting for AIDS prevention efforts among young people, but in some countries social "taboos" have prevented the incorporation of sex education into school curricula. In Trinidad and Tobago, a group

---

Box 3-2. The Health and Family Life Education (HFLE) Initiative in the Caribbean

The HFLE initiative brings together a wide range of diverse partners—the CARICOM Ministers of Education and Health, the University of the West Indies, PAHO/WHO, the U.N. Population Fund (UNFPA), the U.N. Children's Fund (UNICEF), the U.N. International Drug Control Programme (UNDCP), the U.N. Development Programme (UNDP), UNAIDS, and others.

HFLE is implemented through this partnership arrangement and the program provides the basis for a proactive rather than crisis approach to reach young people with information in areas such as HIV/AIDS, sexual health, substance abuse, environmental health, safety and nutrition. Students will be empowered with skills, values, attitudes, and knowledge and will have the opportunity to enact "real life" situations in the classroom; this approach will promote behavior change.

A single plan of action entitled *A Strategy for Strengthening HFLE in CARICOM States* will be implemented by the partner agencies. This initiative has four major challenges: (1) to improve teacher training; (2) to develop comprehensive life skills based teaching materials for HFLE; (3) to strengthen coordination among institutions engaged in HFLE in regional and national levels; and (4) to raise the status of HFLE at all levels of the educational system.

Source: UNAIDS 1999 and EU, 1999.

---

has recently recommended adding a comprehensive HIV/AIDS education program to the curriculum of the nation's secondary schools. The need for such a program was suggested by a 1994 survey among young people ages 12 to 20 that indicated these young people were grossly misinformed about AIDS prevention.

Unfortunately, some children in the Caribbean are forced to drop out of school at an early age. In Haiti, for example, less than half of all children reach the fifth grade. Children who leave school are among the young people at the highest risk of HIV infection, and for beginning of criminal careers. For these children, as well as others, it is important AIDS prevention efforts take place not only in schools, but in shelters, in clinics, in workplaces, in sports clubs, on the street, and wherever young people congregate. Communication—among young people, between children and adults, and within communities—as a whole is essential. Comprehensive approaches that harness the creativity and energy of parents, schools, religious institutions, and the private sector must be used to reach young people in the Caribbean with effective HIV/AIDS prevention messages.

For children who are living on the streets, HIV prevention approaches should include counseling and a broad range of health care and other support services. Campaigns targeting sexually active youth and advising "safer sex" with the use of condoms have been controversial in the Caribbean and elsewhere. Religious leaders could help in AIDS prevention efforts by promoting behaviors among young people such as promoting abstinence and fidelity, which are clearly important.

Nevertheless, realism urges policymakers and educators and other health workers to also provide young people with other means of protecting themselves against HIV infection. Street children who turn to sex for economic survival, for example, are unlikely to respond to calls for abstinence.

Whether in Thailand or Uganda, communities that have adopted a comprehensive approach to the prevention of HIV/AIDS have been rewarded with a lower rate of infection and less stigma and discrimination directed at those living with HIV or AIDS. On the basis of this experience, UNAIDS and its cosponsors have put forward a global strategy featuring seven major sets of action (see Box 3-3).

Box 3-3. UNAIDS Global Strategy for Young People and HIV/AIDS: Seven Steps for Moving Forward

1. Establish or review national policies to reduce the vulnerability of young people to HIV/AIDS and ensure that their rights are respected, protected and fulfilled.

2. Promote young people's genuine participation in expanding national responses to HIV/AIDS.

3. Support peer and youth groups in the community to contribute to local and national responses to HIV/AIDS.

4. Mobilize parents, policymakers, media, and religious organizations to influence public opinions and policies with regard to HIV/AIDS and young people.

5. Improve the quality and coverage of school programs that include HIV/AIDS and related issues.

6. Expand access to youth-friendly health services including HIV/STD prevention, testing and counseling, care and support services.

7. Ensure care and support of orphans and young people living with HIV/AIDS.

Source: UNAIDS, 1999

Programs to prevent sexual transmission of HIV among adults

Caribbean countries have adopted a variety of approaches to preventing the spread of HIV/AIDS among adults. Several Caribbean countries have adopted laws in an effort to prevent the spread of the disease:

- Laws making HIV/AIDS a notifiable disease, for example, have been enacted in Guyana, Jamaica, Saint Lucia, and Belize. Some attorneys argue that Trinidad and Tobago should do the same. They, warn, however, that the legislation should include safeguards regarding the confidentiality of HIV/AIDS tests. Their concern is that once a person's HIV status is known in Trinidad and Tobago, the person's access to services and health insurance declines.

- To reduce discrimination against people with HIV and AIDS, a law in the Dominican Republic specifies the rights of persons infected with HIV and the duties of employers, doctors, and others who interact with such individuals. NGOs are now trying to monitor the law's enforcement.

- Legislation to coerce rapists and sex offenders into HIV testing are in place in the Bahamas and Bermuda, whose HIV/AIDS rates top the regional average. Legislators in Trinidad and Tobago have considered similar legislation.

- In Trinidad and Tobago, a policy paper on HIV/AIDS prepared by legal analysts recommended that the country emphasize an educational approach to preventing HIV/AIDS rather than a legislative approach. Although there is a high degree of awareness of HIV/AIDS in the Caribbean, there is still ignorance and misinformation about what causes AIDS and how to prevent it. Some people in the region still do not even know that using condoms can help prevent AIDS.

Various approaches can be used to educate people about the prevention of HIV/AIDS. Marketing techniques used for selling goods and services can be very effective in reaching out to people to teach them about AIDS. Some Caribbean countries have implemented condom social marketing projects that use a combination of (1) commercial marketing techniques to educate people about the benefits of condoms and (2) commercial distribution channels to sell condoms at subsidized prices. One Caribbean country that is considered a condom social marketing success story, for example, is Haiti. Population Services International implemented a program there that raised people's awareness of the effectiveness of condoms in preventing AIDS and also made condoms available at affordable prices.

Countries with condom social marketing programs and sex worker interventions may want to include and test the female condom (a polyethelene vaginal sheath which women can insert before sex) as an additional option. Women in the Caribbean (and elsewhere) urgently need some method that they can use to protect *themselves* against HIV infection if their male partner does not wish to use condoms. Another option that women could theoretically use to protect themselves from HIV infection is anti-HIV microbicides. Several microbicidal products are currently in clinical testing, and at least two of the products are expected to enter final phase testing in the near future.

Religious institutions represent a major resource in the effort to prevent the spread of HIV/AIDS in the Caribbean. Following the example of the Caribbean Council of Churches, which is engaged as part of the Caribbean Task Force on HIV/AIDS, the creation of forums and formal alliances among the various religious organizations involved in the effort to combat AIDS at the country level ought to be given priority consideration. Such arrangements were recently established in Africa (see Box 3-4).

Businesses are another potential resource in the effort to prevent the spread of HIV/AIDS. The Global Business Council on HIV/AIDS is an association of companies

> **Box 3-4. The International Religious Alliance on HIV/AIDS for Africa**
>
> In June 1999, following a three-day workshop in Senegal, religious leaders and medical experts from various African nations formed a new body to help prevent the spread of HIV/AIDS in Africa: The International Religious Alliance on HIV/AIDS for Africa. The group will be based in Dakar under the auspices of two NGOs involved in AIDS-control work: a Muslim NGO, and a Catholic AIDS services provider. The new body will work closely with scientists in prevention efforts at the grassroots level, and fight the stigmatization of people living with HIV/AIDS through associations of religious leaders to be created in every country.
>
> *Source:* PANA, 1999

committed to the response to AIDS and actively pursuing their own activities in the fight against AIDS, both at and beyond the workplace. Businesses throughout the Caribbean ought to be continuously persuaded that it makes good businesses sense to invest in programs that save their workers and their customers. In countries where sex tourism is common, for example, the Ministries of Tourism and Health should collaborate to identify tour operators that cater specifically to sex tourists and make their activities safe. A regional effort to improve the health and hygiene conditions for guests and staff in Caribbean hotels—the Caribbean Healthy Hotels Project (CHHP)—is being led by PAHO, CAREC, the Caribbean Hotel Association, and Caribbean Action for Sustainable Tourism.

Programs to prevent sexual transmission of HIV by treating STDs

Growing research evidence indicates that common and curable vaginal infections significantly raise a women's risk for HIV infection. For that reason, HIV prevention efforts should include aggressive treatment and screening of STDs for women and their sexual partners. A World Bank report entitled *Safe Motherhood and the World Bank*: *Lessons from 10 Years of Experience* recommends packaging together pregnancy and delivery care, family planning, and management of STDs to achieve the greatest benefit at lowest cost. Given wide-ranging economic, technical, cultural and social constraints, even small steps toward integration of these services can be valuable.

Preventing Mother-to-Child Transmission of HIV

The industrialized world has experienced a decline in the rates of mother-to-child transmission of HIV, but in the developing world, including most of the Caribbean, these rates continue to rise. The widening gap in mother-to-child HIV transmission is due to two things. First, many HIV-positive women in developing countries do not have access to prophylactic drugs that can help prevent HIV transmission during pregnancy and delivery. Second, many HIV-positive women in developing countries breast-feed their babies and thereby transmit HIV to them. Up to one-third of all cases of mother-to-child transmission of HIV are due to breast-feeding.

Providing prophylactic drug therapy to HIV-positive mothers and their newborns

A 1994 clinical trial demonstrated that a particular regimen of the antiviral drug zidovudine (AZT) administered to pregnant women during pregnancy and delivery and to their infants after birth reduced the mother-to-child HIV transmission rate more than 80%. The cost of this particular regimen of AZT—between US$800 and US$900 per woman treated, excluding the costs of voluntary counseling and testing and formula feeding for the infant—is far beyond the capabilities of developing countries in the Caribbean or elsewhere.

Fortunately, however, there may be an alternative. A just-completed study by the Johns Hopkins University School of Medicine suggests that nevirapine (sold as Viramune) proved to be even better than AZT in reducing mother-to-child HIV transmission and at a considerably lower cost (only about $4 per child). Moreover, the low price of nevirapine may attract subsidization by donor and charitable organizations that previously believed they could not make a difference.

Modifying newborn feeding practices

In developing countries, policymakers are struggling to develop appropriate and feasible guidelines on breast-feeding for HIV-positive mothers. By choosing artificial feeding, a woman may avoid passing on HIV to her child, but where the water supply is unsafe, she may also expose her child to other deadly diseases. In some cases, bottle-feeding may even lead to the social ostracism of a woman and her child. The issue is complicated by the fact that few HIV women in developing countries know what their HIV status is.

Several basic research gaps need to be addressed in order to make final recommendations on breast-feeding policy for HIV-positive women in developing countries. One critical area is operational research to study the impact of the use of breast milk substitutes on infant mortality and HIV-infection status.

The screening of donated blood and plasma for HIV antibody began in the Caribbean in 1985. By 1989, all 19 CAREC-reporting countries had the appropriate technology in place and offered a facility for the initial screening of sera for HIV infection. In addition, CAREC established an HIV confirmatory testing service to serve the national laboratories. Since then, laboratories in CAREC countries have gradually established their own confirmatory capabilities. People at high risk of HIV infection have also been encouraged not to donate blood.

The fact that transmission of HIV through blood or blood products accounts for less than 3% of AIDS cases in the Caribbean suggests that more efforts are needed to eliminate this source of infection.

DIAGNOSIS OF HIV/AIDS IN CARIBBEAN COUNTRIES

HIV testing is available in both public and private sector laboratories in the Caribbean. The distribution of public sector laboratories that performed HIV testing in CAREC countries as of 1994 is shown in Table 3-1. By 1997, HIV testing was offered by private sector laboratories in at least 13 CARICOM countries. The distribution of private sector laboratory services was uneven.

By request, CAREC has conducted safety audits and workshops in several national laboratories and has circulated safety guidelines to all national laboratories. Total requests for HIV testing in public sector laboratories rose 44% from 1986 and 1994, and recent trends indicate that the demand for testing will continue to increase.

Table 3-1. Public Sector Health Laboratories That Perform HIV Tests in CAREC Countries, 1994					
Country	Population (1994)	Number of AIDS cases	Total number of labs	Total number of HIV tests	% initially reactive
Anguilla	8,000	0	1	150	0.7
Antigua and Barbuda	65,000	18	1	1,003	15.0
Bahamas, The	272,000	322	2	21,090	7.3
Barbados	261,000	119	1	10,253	2.6
Belize	210,000	18	7	6,845	0.7
Bermuda	63,000	44	2	1,875	1.5
British Virgin Islands	18,000	1	1	971	0.2
Cayman Islands	30,000	3	1	4,955	1.1
Dominica	71,000	5	1	1,439	1.3
Grenada	92,000	7	1	…	…
Guyana	825,000	105	2	5,034	9.9
Jamaica	2,429,000	359	3	31,127	3.1
Montserrat	11,000	0	1	849	1.2
Saint Kitts and Nevis	41,000	5	2	1,932	4.9
Saint Lucia	141,000	13	1	3,652	0.8
Saint Vincent and the Grenadines	111,000	8	1	3,405	0.9
Suriname	418,000	26	2	6,670	0.4*
Trinidad and Tobago	1,292,000	269	2	5,919	14.8
Turks and Caicos Islands	14,000	0	1	2,670	4.2
Total	**6,372,000**	**1,322**	**33**	**109,839**	**4.3**

* Estimate.
…= not available
Source: PAHO/WHO, 1997

CARE AND TREATMENT OF PEOPLE WITH HIV/AIDS IN CARIBBEAN COUNTRIES

The treatment of HIV/AIDS in most Caribbean countries, as in other developing countries, is limited. Public health programs are so under-funded in some countries that health agencies cannot afford inexpensive medications for opportunistic infections such as tuberculosis, much less the thousands of dollars it can cost to treat a single patient with the new combinations of antiviral drugs. A representative of the Caribbean Network for People Living with HIV/AIDS (CRN+) notes that an HIV-positive diagnosis is usually seen as a death sentence in the Caribbean. Infected people and their families need to know that there are options for living available to them. People who are suspected of being HIV-positive are scorned and cast out. The wider community needs more education to combat this stigmatization and discrimination.

Providing Community-Based Care for People with HIV/AIDS

In many Caribbean countries, religious institutions and NGOs are the primary providers of care for people living with HIV/AIDS. In the Dominican Republic, Haiti, and Puerto Rico, for example, hospices and "support houses" run by the Catholic Church provide food, services and pastoral care to young HIV-affected people who have been rejected by their family or community. In addition, there are church-run hospitals for AIDS patients, such as the 120-bed Hospital St Croix de Leoganhe in Haiti, which registers some 24 new HIV-positive cases monthly.

Best practices in family and community care for people with HIV have been captured in a 1999 UNAIDS publication entitled *Comfort and Hope*. One of the six case studies selected was Project Hope, run by a Brazilian NGO, that currently provides services to approximately 480 people living with HIV/AIDS, takes on about 180 new cased per year, and makes about 360 home visit per year, mobilizing a large group of volunteers. These projects provide care and prevention services to people where they live, work, and play. Key commonalties shared by the selected projects include: spiritual motivation or guidance, participation of a well-known community leader, importance of getting moral support of local leaders and authorities, and focus on marginalized groups.

CAREC recently appointed an Ad Hoc Committee on Clinical Management of HIV/AIDS to produce guidelines for the clinical care of individuals infected with HIV that would be applicable to the English-speaking islands of the Caribbean region. The new guidelines, *Clinical Management Guidelines for HIV/AIDS in the Caribbean*, are set at three levels of complexity of care depending on available health facilities. The use of these guidelines is expected to result in a significant improvement in the clinical care of persons infected with HIV in the English-speaking Caribbean.

Treating Tuberculosis—The Leading HIV-Associated Opportunistic Disease

Tuberculosis is the leading HIV-associated opportunistic disease. According to PAHO, most of the reported cases of tuberculosis (TB) in Latin America and the Caribbean occur in people ages 25 to 54. An estimated 30 to 70% of young adults in developing countries are infected with *Mycobacterium tuberculosis*, but the majority will not develop active TB in their lungs. When TB carriers become infected with HIV, however, the virus destroys their immune system, and many more then progress from latent to active TB.

For that reason, countries with high HIV infection rates are experiencing a resurgence of TB. In Haiti and the Dominican Republic, for example, the rates of pulmonary TB are rising alarmingly. In 1998, the incidence of TB in Haiti was 123 per 100,000 population; and the incidence in the Dominican Republic was 51.9 per 100,000 population. Other Caribbean countries have reported rates between 15 and 50, such as Guyana (37.5/100,000), Bahamas (25.4/100,000), Trinidad and Tobago (22.7/100,000), and Suriname (17.9/100,000).

TB can be cured with six to eight months of daily treatment with a combination of antibiotics. To ensure thorough treatment, WHO recommends that TB patients take their antibiotics in the presence of a health or community worker who can observe and supervise the therapy. This approach to the treatment of TB is called DOTS (Directly Observed Treatment, Short course), and by 1999, it has been implemented by many Caribbean countries (e.g., Cuba, Belize, Haiti, Dominican Republic, Guyana, Suriname and English-speaking Caribbean countries). DOTS has universal efficacy, curing TB in 85% of cases; in high burden countries, however, with high HIV prevalence, results are lower even under ideal conditions due to high case fatality rates. In 1997, in Caribbean DOTS countries, such as Haiti, 63.6% of registered patients in DOTS demonstration areas were cured at the end of treatment (PAHO/WHO, 2000). Furthermore, the effective treatment of TB in patients with HIV infection extends these individuals' lives and quickly makes them noncontagious, thus preventing further spread of TB.

Five elements are needed for countries to implement a successful DOTS program (see Box 3-5). By the end of 1998, some 22 countries in the Americas had adopted the DOTS strategy. DOTS pilot areas were recently initiated in several countries, including Brazil, Ecuador, El Salvador, Haiti, Honduras, and Mexico. In 1999, Colombia, the Dominican Republic, Panama, and Paraguay launched the approach. The challenge for these DOTS pilot programs is to gain full support from governments and external partners so that they expand rapidly to have an impact. Success begins with action by communities, but support from the highest levels of government and civil society can make the difference in infectious disease control—as shown with TB control in recent years in the United States and Peru.

Box 3-5. Elements Needed to Implement DOTS for Tuberculosis

Five elements are critical to implementing a successful DOTS (Directly Observed Treatment, Short course) treatment strategy for tuberculosis:

1. Government/political commitment to the tuberculosis control program.

2. Detection of cases, especially in persons who come to the health services with respiratory symptoms, through sputum smear microscopy.

3. Standardized short-course directly observed treatment of all cases with a positive microscopic sputum examination.

4. A regular supply of medicines.

5. A registration and information/monitoring system.

Source: MAP, 1998

The countries of the English-speaking Caribbean in general have not yet carried out a coordinated set of interventions to control TB. On the other hand, the health authorities in the English-speaking Caribbean countries do offer short-course treatment for TB with hospitalization during the first four to six weeks. This regimen probably limits transmission of the TB and allows for the patient's sputum to convert to negative.

New efforts in Africa and Asia can also provide lessons—as well as renewed UNAIDS/WHO collaboration on finding effective models of community-care and early detection of infection and treatment for latent infection and active disease. Working on TB and HIV/AIDS provides opportunities for measuring impact even in the short-run, given the powerful outcome and impact indicators that can be derived from routine health systems data for TB control.

Providing Antiretroviral Drug Therapy for People with HIV/AIDS

Since 1996, triple-combination antiretroviral therapy, a combination of protease inhibitors and anti-HIV drugs, has prolonged the lives and improve the quality of life for thousands of people living with HIV/AIDS in industrialized countries. In general, people who are infected with AIDS in developing countries, including countries in the Caribbean, do not have access to the newer antiretroviral therapies. The cost of the new therapies—at Western market prices of $1,000 per month per patient—is prohibitive for most HIV-infected people in these countries. Moreover, although newer drugs can occasionally be accessed, there is not a consistent and steady supply. For that reason, physicians in developing countries are sometimes reluctant to prescribe the newer drugs.

A 1998 UNAIDS review of access to HIV-related drugs and NGO activities in several countries, including the Dominican Republic, Haiti, and Jamaica, found that none of these countries' governments make antiretroviral treatment available for people with HIV/AIDS. Some NGOs, in these countries—including the PAHO-funded PROMESS (Programme des Medicaments Essentiels) in Haiti and CRN+ in the Dominican Republic and Jamaica—do provide antiretroviral drugs for people with HIV and AIDS, but the supply is uncertain and by no means adequate for the treatment of all those in need.

Recently, UNAIDS and a number of pharmaceutical companies have been testing the feasibility of delivering state-of-the art AIDS treatment in four developing countries—Chile, Uganda, Ivory Coast, and Vietnam. The pilot countries established a national advisory committee to coordinate drug-related policy and a nonprofit clearinghouse to purchase and distribute HIV-related drugs. The pharmaceutical companies, in turn, made available a range of anti-HIV drugs, including antiretrovirals, and virologic services at subsidized prices. One of the lessons of the pilot is that even if the newer antiretroviral drugs are offered at drastically reduced prices, the cost of the medical infrastructure for delivering the drugs is probably prohibitive in these countries.

Many observers have emphasized that that merely lowering the price of AIDS drugs will not solve the international AIDS crisis. For example, Tom Coates, executive director of the University of California at San Francisco AIDS Research Institute, cautions that if drugs are introduced in a population, but not in sufficient quantities, this policy could be disastrous, making people sicker, rather than better and increasing the possibility for development of drug-resistant HIV strains. He and other public health practitioners working in developing countries have warned that unrealistic expectations of the expensive antiretroviral drug combinations in resource-poor countries may undermine prevention efforts by encouraging the mistaken impression that scientists have found a "cure" for AIDS. The excitement over promising results from trials of new anti-HIV drugs should not obscure prevention—still the most effective approach against the virus.

A few international efforts have been made to provide guidelines for antiretroviral treatment in developing countries. In May 1998 the International AIDS Economics Network sponsored an online conference entitled *Anti-Retroviral Treatment in Developing Countries: Questions of Economics, Equity and Ethics.*

Prospects for the Development of an AIDS Vaccine

Some observers, noting that the antiretroviral drug therapies available to people with HIV/AIDS in the United States and Europe are still too expensive for those in the developing world, have called for increased efforts to develop an AIDS vaccine. There are still difficult scientific, political, and financial obstacles to overcome in the development of an AIDS vaccine. Furthermore, there is no certainty that a vaccine which will be suitable, effective, and affordable in developing countries will be developed in the foreseeable future.

Just as the hope for improved access to costly AIDS drugs should not undermine a strong and unrelenting effort to prevent HIV transmission in developing countries through existing preventive measures, neither should the hope of an AIDS vaccine. At best a vaccine may be a valuable future addition to the set of interventions. *Only strong preventive measures will change the increasing trend in the number of HIV infections in the Caribbean and other developing countries.*

The World Bank recently launched an AIDS Vaccine Task Force to consider how it could speed up development of an AIDS vaccine that is effective and affordable in developing countries. The EU has established a similar task force. These efforts complement the overall HIV vaccine efforts coordinated by UNAIDS with leadership of WHO. In August 1999, the World Bank's AIDS Vaccine Task Force convened a meeting of senior policymakers, donors, and NGOs who met in New Delhi. Participants urged the World Bank to continue efforts to stimulate the development and financing of an AIDS vaccine for low-income countries. They noted that achieving these goals will require the combined efforts of national and international scientists, UNAIDS, WHO, the International AIDS Vaccine Initiative, bilateral organizations, private industry, developing country governments, NGOs, and the World Bank. Similar meetings were held in Brazil and South Africa.

More recently, the World Bank has become an active member of the Global Alliance for Vaccines and Immunizations (GAVI) that is exploring ways of accelerating development of an AIDS vaccine for developing countries. GAVI is a network comprising interested governments, UNICEF, WHO, bilateral agencies, the Gates Foundation, the Rockefeller Foundation and other partners to complement the work of the International AIDS Vaccines Initiative (IAVI).

Intensifying National Responses to HIV/AIDS in the Caribbean: Five Key Steps

As a subregion comprised of small island developing states and mainland nations with relatively- small populations, HIV/AIDS presents unique challenges and the response to it must consider consequences specific to small country circumstances. First, while trends in African countries have suggested that the economic impact of the HIV epidemic becomes evident after experiencing a national HIV seroprevalence of around 7%, such might not be the case with countries with total populations ranging from 100 ,000 to the low millions. In these smaller countries, there is not the population size that might somehow absorb a certain level of the burden before it is significantly evidenced by economic impacts. Second, island communities are often perceived as being challenged with greater confidentiality concerns and breaches than larger countries. Third, the laws and cultural customs inherited through slavery, colonization and other socio- historical phenomena may encourage discrimination and stigmatization of the HIV epidemic and those living with HIV/AIDS or those perceived to be most at risk or vulnerable. Last, providing resources and infrastructures for a comprehensive response to HIV/AIDS in each country might be both resource- prohibitive for each nation, but might also not be realistic in light of the population movement, service delivery and service access patterns in the subregion. Therefore, despite many lessons learned from other country experiences, the Caribbean must learn how to adapt such information to meet the unique needs of its member states.

Building an effective national response to the HIV/AIDS epidemic in the Caribbean would require an enabling environment and the necessary resources to bring proven interventions quickly up to nationwide scale. Although many Caribbean governments have initiated a limited response to HIV/AIDS, much remains to be done to bring the response to the scale necessary. Governments of all Caribbean countries (with their partners) need to expand and intensify their responses rapidly, and to address HIV/AIDS as a multisectoral development issue—not only a health concern. At the national level, the following five actions are fundamental:

- Increasing the national government's commitment, attention, and funding to combat the HIV/AIDS epidemic, including the integration of HIV/AIDS prevention and control into poverty reduction strategies.

- Scaling up prevention activities at the national and community levels.

- Scaling up care activities at the national and community levels.

- Supporting more research at the national level.

- Strengthening regional responses to the epidemic in the Caribbean.

Step 1: Increase the National Government's Commitment, Attention, and Funding Related to HIV/AIDS

Caribbean governments need to expand and intensify their responses to HIV/AIDS rapidly. Many governments in the Caribbean region have not made HIV/AIDS a policy priority. Not all government leaders are convinced of the potential impact of AIDS. Others see the threat but are reluctant to address the issue. Strong government commitment has proved essential in every country that has made headway against the HIV/AIDS epidemic. Given spread of HIV/AIDS in the Caribbean and its impact on the region's economic and social indicators, it is vital that national leaders in the Caribbean region turn their full attention to the challenges of the epidemic. High-level support and political commitment will be crucial to the long-term success of any national or regional effort.

Caribbean governments also need to recognize that HIV/AIDS is a multisectoral development issue—not only a health concern—that requires a multisectoral national program with adequate funding. Moving beyond the Ministries of Health and AIDS-specific NGOs to include representatives of a broad range of other sectors of society in national strategic planning is essential. One major issue that will have to be addressed is how best to allocate scarce resources in light of the rapidly growing costs of AIDS. In developing strategic plans, Caribbean countries should re-examine their spending priorities and allocate their expenditures accordingly. In many cases, they may be able to leverage existing programs (e.g., education, agricultural extension) by integrating HIV/AIDS programs into them at modest cost. Management of national programs should involve the highest office of government to ensure the power, resources, flexibility, and effective coordination to act across sectors.

Step 2: Scale Up HIV/AIDS Prevention Activities

Caribbean governments and their partners need to expand proven interventions to a scale large enough to reach all vulnerable individuals. Given scarce resources, they should focus on a core set of prevention activities that have proven effective and feasible, including the following:

- Communications that move audiences from awareness of HIV/AIDS to risk-reducing behavior.

- Making condoms, the treatment of STDs, and voluntary counseling and testing for HIV more accessible.

- Ensuring a safe blood supply.

- Reducing mother-to-child transmission of HIV.

To ensure effectiveness, governments need to work in partnership with persons living with HIV/AIDS, community groups, religious organizations, NGOs, health professionals, and the private sector. Communities and NGOs need to receive direct financial support to act at the local level, where the public sector is often less effective.

Step 3: Scale Up HIV/AIDS Care Activities

Strategies to provide high-quality community and home-based care need to be developed in Caribbean countries. In addition, Caribbean governments and their partners need to mount programs to care for the thousands of orphans and other vulnerable children whose extended families can no longer bear the full load.

Local NGOs are providing care and treatment for persons living with HIV/AIDS in some countries, including Haiti, the Dominican Republic, and Jamaica. Typically, the NGO sector has expanded partly in response to the growing deficiencies in HIV/AIDS care activities within the public health sector. NGOs are particularly active in Haiti, providing 60-70% of health services in 1996. In the other Caribbean countries, NGOs complement government and for-profit services mostly though health promotion activities. Generally, there has been limited coordination or regulation of the NGOs' programs.

Step 4: Support More Research on HIV/AIDS

Continued research is needed into the cost of HIV/AIDS treatment and care alternatives, the sectoral impact and costs of the epidemic, and the effectiveness of existing tools in different cultural and infrastructure settings. Leaders in each sector of a country's economy will continue to view HIV/AIDS as a health issue unless they see the potential impact on their sector and the relatively low cost of intervention at an early stage.

Step 5: Strengthen the Regional Response to HIV/AIDS in the Caribbean

Regional responses to HIV/AIDS in the Caribbean are discussed in the next chapter. One exciting development is the recent approval by National AIDS Program Directors of *Caribbean Regional Strategic Plan of Action for HIV/AIDS,1999-2004*, developed by the CARICOM-led Caribbean Task Force on HIV/AIDS. If the plan succeeds, there will be an increased pool of personnel able to contribute to effective policy development and implementation of programs in the Caribbean; increased regional awareness of the benefits, costs and operational feasibility of interventions to reduce mother-to-child transmission of HIV; an expanded and effective regional network of people living with HIV/AIDS advocating for improved care and support, and contributing to national policy development; improved regional capacity to design, implement and evaluate interventions to reduce high-risk behavior related to the spread of HIV infection; more comprehensive and accurate information on the course, consequences and costs of the epidemic through improved surveillance, monitoring and evaluation of national control programs and through operational research.

"Every day, we must balance our fears about AIDS against the certain knowledge that human action can make a difference."

Peter Piot, Executive Director of the Joint United Nations Program on HIV/AIDS, "The UNAIDS Report," June 1999

IV REGIONAL RESPONSES TO HIV/AIDS IN THE CARIBBEAN

RATIONALE FOR A REGIONAL RESPONSE TO HIV/AIDS IN THE CARIBBEAN

Strong arguments can be made in support of mounting a more effective regional response to HIV/AIDS in the Caribbean. First, although all of the Caribbean countries have established broad-based, multisectoral National AIDS Committees and taken some measures to control the HIV/AIDS epidemic, the scope and effectiveness of the response has varied considerably, as discussed in Chapter III. Several problems have hampered national efforts to reduce the spread of HIV/AIDS in Caribbean countries. Most of the countries in the Caribbean region are too small to develop alone the capacity to produce the public goods needed to respond to the HIV/AIDS epidemic in the region. In Haiti and Guyana and, to a lesser extent, the Dominican Republic. lack of infrastructure, poverty, and large size have hampered efforts. Another problem in Haiti, which was affected very early in the HIV/AIDS epidemic, has been political instability.

Second, HIV/AIDS is a clearly regional issue. The weak institutional capacity of Haiti, the Dominican Republic, and Guyana to respond to the HIV/AIDS, for example, is a problem that transcends national boundaries because many HIV-positive people have left these countries in search of support and care in better off communities elsewhere in the Caribbean region. Strengthening regional institutions and networks would enable all countries in the region, even the smallest, to benefit.

Third, the HIV/AIDS epidemic is a long-term problem demanding a sustained response by qualified health care and other personnel, which many countries lack. The response to HIV/AIDS in the Caribbean currently depends on too few qualified and informed individuals. There is no systematic teaching at the postgraduate level of communication approaches that will get people to alter their sexual behavior. Only scant attention is paid to issues involved in treating STDs and caring for people with HIV/AIDS in the curricula used to train doctors and nurses in the Caribbean. Health economics is also a poorly developed discipline in the Caribbean. Policy analysis and development is carried out in an environment largely isolated from global policy information.

Finally, opportunities exist for concerted regional action to make HIV/AIDS a priority development issue that transcends party politics, points to shared interests, and encourages commitment to take on shared vulnerabilities and responsibilities, especially related to sustaining political will and enacting national policies that address human rights and legal and ethical issues related to HIV/AIDS.

INTERNATIONAL DONORS' ACTIVITIES RELATED TO HIV/AIDS IN THE CARIBBEAN

UNAIDS and Its Co-Sponsors' Activities

UNAIDS—which is co-sponsored by UNICEF, UNDCP, UNDP, UNFPA, UNESCO, WHO, and the World Bank—is the leading advocate for worldwide action against HIV/AIDS. The largest donors to UNAIDS in 1998 were the governments of the United States, the Netherlands, the United Kingdom, and the Scandinavian countries. With an annual budget of US$60 million, the UNAIDS Secretariat operates as a catalyst and coordinator of action on AIDS rather than as a direct funding or implementing agency.

UNAIDS Caribbean office in Port-of-Spain, Trinidad, works with a broad array of partners in the Caribbean—including National AIDS Programs, CARICOM, CAREC, the European Community, NGOs, and others. UNAIDS' and its co-sponsors' current commitments/disbursements in Latin America and the Caribbean are about 5 million Euros. Among UNAIDS co-sponsors, PAHO/WHO provides the most support to the Caribbean region. Most of PAHO's support in the Caribbean region has been provided for the work of CAREC, a specialized agency of PAHO. UNICEF is active in supporting the CARICOM-led Health and Family Life Education (HFLE) Program (see Chapter III) and the integration of HIV/AIDS interventions in that program. UNDP is exploring ways to increase its support to the Caribbean's efforts to confront the development impacts and consequences of HIV/AIDS. In March 1999, UNDP held the First Caribbean Workshop on HIV and Development in Barbados.

Over half of the 5 million Euros in funding provided by UNAIDS and its co-sponsors is to improve the U.N. System's response to HIV/AIDS and to support inter-country U.N. advisory services. Areas of UNAIDS assistance include strategic planning exercises, resource mobilization, political networking, capacity building, strengthening networks of persons living with HIV/AIDS, strengthening technical cooperation between countries of the region, and funding specific interventions (e.g., to prevent mother-to-child HIV transmission, AIDS management, peer education, tourism, female condom social marketing). UNAIDS' support is also provided for studies of HIV voluntary counseling and testing, communication programs, and ways to strengthen horizontal cooperation among Caribbean countries to improve national response capacities.

European Union and Canada

The European Union (EU) is the major external financier of a response to HIV/AIDS in the Caribbean, having committed or disbursed over 11 million Euros to date. Significant support has been made available from EU special budget-lines and the Economic Development Fund (EDF) for HIV prevention interventions in Haiti (1 million Euros), the Dominican Republic (1.96 million Euros), Trinidad and Tobago (550,000 Euros), Suriname (891,000 Euros), Guyana (850,000 Euros), and Grenada, (569,000 Euros). Smaller amounts have been made available from the EDF to strengthen STD diagnostic and HIV testing capabilities in Antigua and Barbuda, St. Lucia, St. Vincent and the Grenadines, the Turks and Caicos Islands, Barbados, and St. Kitts and Nevis.

Within the English-speaking Caribbean, international donor support for regional initiatives in the fight against HIV/AIDS has generally been channeled over the years through CAREC. Here, France (FTC), Germany (GTZ), and Canada (CIDA) have funneled their support to more traditional public health efforts of blood safety, the prevention of HIV transmission via condoms and STD control, and the use of mass media or other communications to help prevent the spread of HIV/AIDS.

The EU is pose to begin a major new initiative to assist CARICOM member states in responding to issues pertaining to HIV/AIDS and population mobility (including tourism): *Strengthening the Institutional Response to HIV/AIDS in the Caribbean Project* (see Box 4-1). Developed in consultation with UNAIDS, the Inter-American Development Bank (IADB), PAHO, people living with HIV/AIDS, and others, the project, which has not yet been approved, will last about three years and cost 6.425 million Euros. It involves six regional institutions—CARICOM, CAREC, CRN+, UNAIDS, the Caribbean Research Council, and the University of the West Indies—and 24 countries. It also places the EU (together with USAID in Haiti, the Dominican Republic, Guyana and Jamaica) in the position of being the major donor to regional HIV/AIDS activities in the Caribbean. An unquantifiable but important contribution will be made to the project by CARICOM member states, which make annual contributions to CARICOM, the University of the West Indies, and CAREC.

The Strengthening the Institutional Response to HIV/AIDS in the Caribbean Project represents an important contribution to an expanded and sustained response to HIV/AIDS in the Caribbean and has potentially large development benefits. The EU-funded project will offer technical, material, and financial support to regional institutions to expand and improve their response to HIV/AIDS so that the effectiveness and sustainability of national interventions in the Caribbean region improves. Specifically, the project will aim to do the following: (1) support accurate and complete data collection on the incidence and prevalence of HIV/AIDS in all countries in the Caribbean; (2) assist policymakers in at least 10 countries of the Caribbean to use public health economic analysis to inform decisions to allocate funds to HIV/AIDS ; (3) support the inclusion of modules in behavior change communication, health economics, and care of people with HIV/AIDS in postgraduate studies in HIV/AIDS at the University of the West Indies; and (4) empower people with HIV to be actively involved in key policymaking bodies (National AIDS Committees/Programs) in half of the countries in the Caribbean region.

CARICOM will help to implement the EU-funded project *Strengthening the Institutional Response to HIV/AIDS in the Caribbean* under an agreement with CARIFORUM, a regional institution set up to coordinate EU regional projects. The project will be implemented in all Caribbean countries that are members of CARIFORUM. Since the project spans over many countries and six regional institutions, its implementation will require continual consultation. A considerable amount of money has been budgeted for regional consultation and consensus-building.

U.S. Agency for International Development (USAID) Activities

USAID has sponsored HIV/AIDS prevention programs in the Caribbean region for over a decade through two Washington-funded cooperative agreements with Family Health International. Under one agreement, from 1991 to 1997, Family Health International implemented the AIDS Control and Prevention (AIDSCAP) in 45 countries, including the Dominican Republic, Haiti, and Jamaica.

Box 4-1. Overview of the Proposed European Union-Funded Project:
Strengthening the Institutional Response to HIV/AIDS in the Caribbean

The EU recently committed to fund a major new project to assist CARICOM Member States in responding to issues pertaining to HIV/AIDS. The project has not yet finally approved.

- *Strengthening the Caribbean region's capacity to develop policies for reducing the incidence of HIV/AIDS:* With the proposed role of CARICOM, and in particular with the establishment of its Human and Social Development Council, the Caribbean region is said to have the infrastructure to develop and carry forward regional approaches to region-wide problems. Given the history and experience of the previous Ministerial Councils, there is every reason to believe that these structures need support to become effective.

  The EU-funded project will address this issue by providing institutional support to CARICOM, encouraging inter-country exchanges and the greater involvement of people with HIV/AIDS in policy formulation. The involvement of UNAIDS in providing access to global policy development and information on program "best practice" is also important. For too long, the Caribbean region has been developing HIV/AIDS policy in isolation from, and sometimes at variance with, international policy.

- *Strengthening the Caribbean region's capacity to develop and implement HIV/AIDS programs:* Capacity to develop and implement HIV/AIDS interventions varies across the Caribbean region. In Jamaica, the evidence appears to suggest that an early and sustained multisectoral STD control program has been effective in stemming the spread of HIV. In some countries, lack of government commitment and action has allowed the epidemic to spread to the general population. Building national capacity to respond to the epidemic requires short-term support, and long term sustained investment in human resource development.

  For that reason, the EU-funded project will support the expansion of existing programs, such as CAREC's activity in surveillance and program development, as well as longer term investments in capacity building, such as those in training and economic analysis at the University of the West Indies, and in policy development, through support to CARICOM, CRN+, and UNAIDS. The implementation of policy will depend on the motivation that exists at the national level. The existence of broad-based, multisectoral National AIDS Committees in every country reflects an already high level of motivation. The limitation on these organizations is mainly one of isolation from international policy and lack of resources and it is in this area the present EU-funded project aims to make a difference.

- *Availability of capacity for addressing the HIV/AIDS epidemic in both the public and private sectors:* In all the Caribbean countries, the public sector has taken the lead in mounting some form of response to the HIV/AIDS problem. In some countries, however, the private sector, especially insurance companies, trade unions, and employers' associations, have begun to express the desire for inclusion in policy discussions related to the problem. What is needed is a division of labor between the public and private sectors so that capacity expansion will take place in a complementary manner. It is hoped that the effort to create National Business Councils on HIV/AIDS as part of the present EU-funded project will contribute to this particular goal.

- *Justification of the investment:* Although it is not unreasonable to expect a private market for the treatment of STDs to emerge if disposable incomes are large enough, the private sector will not normally take the lead in the provision of public goods such as preventive services, policy and epidemiological research, and behavior-change information. This is why public and quasi-public institutions must be relied upon to reduce the incidence of HIV/AIDS. When at the national level such institutions are faced with fiscal pressures and uncertainties it makes sense to have the required interventions mediated through a regional institution. Institutions like CARICOM, CAREC, and the University of the West Indies provides a genuine opportunity for sensible investments aimed at addressing HIV/AIDS.

  On another level, the justification of the proposed investment in bringing about a reduction in the incidence of HIV/AIDS in the region lies in the latest estimate of the economic impact of HIV/AIDS on two countries where studies have been done, Trinidad and Tobago and Jamaica. Estimates suggest that this will amount to more than 400 million Euros annually by the year 2000 if no successful intervention takes place. A European Community investment of 6.367 million Euros has a potentially very large cost-benefit ratio.

- *Efficiency of the investment:* In respect of the efficiency of the investment, most prevention strategies involve the production of public goods. Financing through non-private sources, preferably ones which do not incur an excess burden via taxation, is justified. Since project financing falls into this category of funding the efficiency argument is adequately made. Source: EU, 1999.

- The only alternatives to project activities in an effort to reduce the impacts of HIV/AIDS are a preventive vaccine, a cure for the disease, or effective and affordable treatments. Vaccines are now only in the experimental stage and to date there is no cure. Treatments are available, but their long-term efficacy and safety is uncertain and their cost significant (to treat the 18,000 people with HIV/AIDS in the Caribbean with antiretroviral therapies would cost about 360 million Euros a year, or 1140 million Euros over the life of the EU-funded project). In this sense, the project will support the only known ways of achieving the goal of reducing the spread of HIV/AIDS.

Source: EU, 1999.

Under a second agreement, Family Health International is implementing the Implementing AIDS Care and Prevention (IMPACT) Project, now in its first year, in 25 countries, including Dominican Republic and Jamaica. The AIDS Communications Project (AIDSCOM) of the Academy of Educational Development (AED) also provided support for HIV/AIDS education and information in the early response to HIV/AIDS and provided resident adviser assistance to some Caribbean countries.

In the Dominican Republic, Haiti, and Jamaica, USAID currently provides about US$6 million in support to the national STD/HIV/AIDS program, NGOs, and other private sector groups. USAID has supported the Haitian Government's response to HIV/AIDS through the Health Systems 2004 project, which focuses on condom social marketing, voluntary counseling and testing for HIV, and strategic planning. Funding for Guyana (US$600,000 per year) for the next three years is expected by the year 2000. USAID at one time supported CAREC's Special Program on Sexually Transmitted Infections (see discussion below) but discontinued its involvement in 1994.

CARIBBEAN REGIONAL ORGANIZATIONS' HIV/AIDS-RELATED INITIATIVES

The Secretariat of the CARICOM is the organization responsible for regional policy and cooperation in the Caribbean region, and its Human and Social Development Division has assumed a lead role in regional HIV/AIDS initiatives in the Caribbean. Two other regional organizations that have been involved in such initiatives are CAREC and the Caribbean Network of People with HIV/AIDS (CRN+). CARICOM, CAREC, and CRN+ are three of the six institutions that will be implementing the EU-s new project *Strengthening the Institutional Response to HIV/AIDS in the Caribbean* discussed earlier.

CARICOM Initiatives

The Secretariat of the CARICOM is the organization responsible for regional policy and cooperation in the Caribbean region, and its Human and Social Development Division has assumed a lead role in regional HIV/AIDS initiatives in the Caribbean. As mentioned in Chapter III, for example, CARICOM has played a lead role in the implementation of the Health and Family Life Education (HFLE) program—the goal of which is to proactively provide young people in the Caribbean region with information on HIV/AIDS, sexual health, substance abuse, environmental health, safety, and nutrition.

In June 1998, UNAIDS, CARICOM, and the EU jointly organized a pan-Caribbean Consultation on HIV/AIDS involving 22 countries and territories, as well as regional and international partners. That meeting underscored the need for a well-coordinated, multisectoral expanded response to the HIV/AIDS epidemic in the Caribbean and resulted in the establishment of the Caribbean Task Force on HIV/AIDS, with a formal mandate from the Ministers of Health of the participating countries to coordinate and strengthen the regional response to the HIV/AIDS epidemic.

The Caribbean Task Force on HIV/AIDS is chaired by the CARICOM Secretariat. Members include national experts in key HIV/AIDS programming areas, the Caribbean Network for People Living with HIV/AIDS (CRN+), UNAIDS, CAREC, PAHO/WHO, UNICEF, UNDP, the University of the West Indies, the EU, the Caribbean Development Bank, the Inter-American Development Bank, the World Bank, Caribbean Council of Churches, the Association of Caribbean States, the Caribbean Tourism Organization, the Commonwealth Youth Program, the

Caribbean News Agency, the Caribbean Congress of Labor, and many other representatives of civil society. Recently, the Caribbean Task Force on HIV/AIDS led a wide consultative process and developed a comprehensive strategic plan for the region. That plan, the *Caribbean Regional Strategic Plan of Action for HIV/AIDS, 1999-2004,* is discussed at length in the concluding section of this chapter.

CAREC Initiatives

CAREC, a specialized agency affiliated with PAHO, is the institution in the Caribbean region that has the longest experience responding substantively to the HIV/AIDS epidemic. CAREC's Special Program on Sexually Transmitted Infections has for many years encouraged the involvement of multiple sectors in the fight against HIV/AIDS in the English- and Dutch-speaking Caribbean countries.

CAREC's Special Program on Sexually Transmitted Infections has been almost wholly externally financed. France provided a grant to CAREC of 650,000 Euros that comes to an end in December 2000. Germany is providing CAREC with 1.6 million Euros for general support, possibly to be renewed. Canada has provided a grant of 2.6 million Euros of support to CAREC's Special Program that ends in early 2001.

CRN+ Initiatives

CRN+ , an organization established in 1996, is based in Trinidad and Tobago but has affiliates in 17 countries in the Caribbean region. Its goals are to share information, build capacity among persons living with HIV/AIDS, and support HIV/AIDS advocacy in the countries of the Caribbean. CRN+ is a member of the Caribbean Task Force on HIV/AIDS and. CRN+ has received support from the United Nations Volunteers to its regional office and to assist in building networks in five countries. They will receive significant institutional development support through the new EU project as one of the six institutions implementing that project.

THE CARIBBEAN REGIONAL STRATEGIC PLAN OF ACTION FOR HIV/AIDS, 1999-2004: A REGIONAL FRAMEWORK FOR COLLABORATION

As noted previously, the Caribbean Task Force on HIV/AIDS was established in June 1998 with a mandate to coordinate and strengthen the regional response to the HIV/AIDS epidemic in the Caribbean. Through a broad consultative process, the Task Force has worked with National AIDS Program Coordinators representing virtually all of the Caribbean countries and territories, it developed the *Caribbean Regional Strategic Plan of Action for HIV/AIDS, 1999-2000. It* includes six major areas for regional action: (1) advocacy, policy development, and legislation; (2) care and support of people living with HIV/AIDS; (3) prevention of HIV transmission in young people; (4) prevention of HIV transmission among vulnerable populations; (5) prevention of mother to child transmission of HIV; and (6) strengthening national and regional response capabilities (see Table 4-1).

Table 4-1. Caribbean Regional Strategic Plan of Action for HIV/AIDS, 1999-2004:
Priority Areas and Strategic Actions

Priority Areas for Action	Strategic Actions
1. Advocacy, Policy Development, and Legislation	Promote human rights and nondiscrimination Target leadership in critical sectors HIV/AIDS and health reform Conduct research on impacts Conduct vaccine trials
2. Care and Support of People Living with HIV/AIDS	Conduct situational analysis on access and quality of care Develop regional standards of care Extend counseling and diagnostic facilities Extend networks of persons living with HIV/AIDS and support them
3. Prevention of HIV Transmission Among Young People	Support the implementation of the Health and Family Life Education (HFLE) initiative Integrate into adolescent programs, including reproductive health programs Condom promotion Research and innovation in methodology Peer counseling Sexual health education for youth in and out of school
4. Prevention of HIV Transmission Among Vulnerable Populations: • Men having sex with men • Sex workers • Drug users • Institutionalized populations • Uniformed populations • Mobile populations (e.g., migrant workers, sex workers, tourists)	Support development of regional networks Support research and development to define best practices Support implementation of UNDCP plan of action Integrate HIV/AIDS prevention and care into prison health care programs Targeted information, education, and communication (IEC) programs Conduct situational analyses Include HIV/AIDS issues in tourism and health initiatives Develop regional policy and operational guidelines Identify and support field training sites/models
5. Prevention of Mother-to-Child HIV Transmission	Target women for IEC programs Negotiate with pharmaceutical companies for access to antiviral drugs for prevention of mother-to-child HIV transmission Close collaboration with UNICEF for program development and implementation
6. Strengthening Regional and National Response Capabilities	Network with regional agencies and NGOs Support capacity building in key agencies Upgrade HIV/AIDS surveillance Develop a comprehensive IEC strategy and program Develop research agenda and promote implementation Promote technical cooperation among countries Develop coordinated approach to resource mobilization Target the private sector Strengthen monitoring and evaluation capacity

Source: CARICOM/Caribbean Task Force on HIV/AIDS, 2000.

The National AIDS Program Directors met in Antigua in June 1999 to review and approve the draft regional strategic plan, and the final version of the plan was published in February 2000. The implementation of the five-year strategic plan will be overseen by the Caribbean Task Force on HIV/AIDS under CARICOM's leadership. The activities called for in the plan will be financed largely through existing programs and projects, including the new EU-funded project that focuses on strengthening the institutional response to HIV/AIDS (see discussion above). If necessary, the Caribbean Task Force on HIV/AIDS will work with the CARICOM Secretariat to mobilize additional resources through multilateral cooperation agreements, the private sector, and UNAIDS resource mobilization mechanisms.

The *Caribbean Regional Strategic Plan of Action for HIV/AIDS, 1999-2004*, lays the groundwork for an expanded and coordinated regional response to the HIV/AIDS epidemic in the Caribbean and provides guidance to Caribbean countries for the design and implementation of more effective national AIDS programs. If the plan succeeds, there will be an increased pool of personnel able to contribute to effective policy development and implementation of programs in the Caribbean; increased regional awareness of the benefits, costs and operational feasibility of interventions to reduce mother-to-child transmission of HIV; an expanded and effective regional network of people living with HIV/AIDS advocating for improved care and support, and contributing to national policy development; improved regional capacity to design, implement and evaluate interventions to reduce high-risk behavior related to the spread of HIV infection; more comprehensive and accurate information on the course, consequences and costs of the epidemic through improved surveillance, monitoring, and evaluation of national control programs and through operational research.

The *Caribbean Regional Strategic Plan of Action for HIV/AIDS, 1999-2004*, provides a clear framework for coordinated action to halt the spread of HIV/AIDS in the Caribbean, and it has been sanctioned by all of the regional institutions and international agencies working in HIV/AIDS in the region. The success of this initiative will hinge on the continuous commitment of leaders of the Caribbean countries to collaborate on this CARICOM-led regional effort. Since the financing for the plan will come largely through existing program and projects, it will also depend on the commitment of the EU, the World Bank, and other international donors. The next chapter discusses the potential role of the World Bank in efforts to prevent and control HIV/AIDS in the Caribbean.

"We must shine a spotlight on the AIDS issue, put it front and center. Break the silence; destigmatize it. And build coalitions with governments, the private sector and civil society to fight it. We must find innovative ways to make care and treatment available, including affordable drugs."

James Wolfensohn, "War on AIDS," Appearance by World Bank President before U.N. Security Council, January 10, 2000

V THE WORLD BANK'S ROLE

WHAT HAS BEEN DONE BY THE WORLD BANK?

The World Bank began providing funding for AIDS prevention in 1986 as part of broader health and sector projects. It began funding free-standing AIDS projects in 1989. In Latin America, World Bank-funded projects in Brazil, Argentina and Haiti aimed to stem the spread of AIDS and STDs in these countries and to prevent it from spreading more broadly in the general population (see Box 5-1).

Box 5-1. Examples of World Bank-Funded AIDS and STD Control Projects in Brazil, Argentina, and Haiti

The following World Bank-funded projects were designed to help curb the spread of AIDS and STDs in these countries and to prevent these diseases from spreading more broadly in the general population.

- *Brazil:* In 1993, the World Bank approved a loan of $160 million for Brazil's AIDS and STD Control Project, which focuses largely on prevention efforts, but also covers treatment, testing, and increasing the government's capacity to deliver services. With the help of about 120 NGOs, the Brazilian Government launched AIDS prevention programs targeting high-risk groups such as injecting-drug users throughout the country. The government was able to expand testing for HIV and other STDs, as well as to introduce 36 new laboratories able to test for HIV. Training programs under the project allowed government staff who diagnose and deliver AIDS services to strengthen their capacity to deal with the epidemic and improve the treatment of patients with HIV and AIDS.

- *Argentina:* In 1998, the World bank approved a loan for US$15 million to promote health and disease prevention activities in Buenos Aires and in the provinces of Cordoba and Santa Fe, where 85% of Argentina's AIDS-related cases are concentrated. This project is increasing the availability of existing diagnostic treatment and counseling services in targeted areas and supporting HIV- and STD-related research and development. It will be implemented with the help of civil society organizations, the Catholic Church, NGOs, trade unions, schools, and student organizations.

- *Haiti:* Under the ongoing First Health Project, support is being provided to boost the national TB, STDs and HIV/AIDS programs, as follows: (i) interventions to increase utilization of TB treatment services; (ii) IEC activities and condom distribution to prevent transmission; (iii) epidemiologic surveillance for STDs and HIV/AIDS; (iv) staff training to improve testing, counseling, and STDs treatment; and (v) program management at the central and department levels.

Source: World Bank data.

The World Bank is one of the leading financiers of HIV/AIDS activities in the world, having committed over US$988.5 million worldwide for 80 ongoing and future projects to prevent and control the spread of HIV/AIDS since 1986. This, however, has not been enough given the scope of the epidemic. The World Bank's loans for HIV/AIDS prevention and control in Brazil and Argentina (two to the Brazilian government and one to the government of Argentina) total US$340 million. Although the Argentina and Brazil loans are on IBRD terms, most of the World Bank's financing for HIV/AIDS-related projects in developing countries is provided on highly concessional terms through the International Development Association.

In addition to providing loans, through the Development Grant Facility, the World Bank provides grants for regional initiatives that tackle the HIV/AIDS epidemic. In Africa and Asia, for example, the World Bank has supported initiatives aimed at strengthening regional cooperation and improving the capacity for neighboring countries to consult on policy and implementation issues. The World Bank has also promoted a regional AIDS Initiative for Latin America and the Caribbean. This initiative— patterned along lines of the initiatives in Africa and Asia and known as SIDALAC—is now being integrated into UNAIDS' regional technical support efforts. SIDALAC is currently focusing on (1) the epidemiology and economic impact of the HIV/AIDS epidemic in Latin America and the Caribbean; (2) the development of interventions to raise awareness of key decision-makers; and (3) the development of innovative interventions in the private sector. SIDALAC has funded the only HIV/AIDS economic impact study in the Caribbean to date, a study that was conducted by the University of the West Indies in collaboration with the CAREC.

The World Bank has recently adopted a new strategic approach to addressing the devastating consequences of HIV/AIDS on development. This approach builds on the important HIV/AIDS-related work that the World Bank and UNAIDS have started and uses these organizations' strong comparative advantages to rapidly increase the level of action and available resources needed to bring up to scale the interventions that can slow the HIV/AIDS epidemic.

As discussed in the World Bank's 1999 publication *Responding to the Crisis: The Intensified Action Against HIV/AIDS in Africa, the World,* the new approach does the following:

- Places countries in the driver's seat to set the course of their response to HIV/AIDS, emphasizing the important role government leadership plays in developing, implementing, and sustaining a multisectoral effort to fight against AIDS, while also noting the importance of partnership with civil society and the private sector.

- Treats AIDS as a priority development issue for the World Bank that impacts upon all sectors and is addressed throughout the Comprehensive Development Framework—a holistic approach that focuses on integrating HIV/AIDS related activities in a multisectoral manner.

- Focuses efforts on protecting new generations, while caring for those already infected and affected by HIV/AIDS.

- Focuses on bringing successful interventions to a national or regional scale, reaching the vulnerable women, youth and rural populations that have not been reached in the past.

- Proposes immediate response by integrating prevention and mitigation efforts into ongoing World Bank projects.

- Specifies concrete actions, with estimated costs, which the World Bank can help countries to undertake.

- Emphasizes building national capacity to respond, supporting country-based responses and decentralized efforts.

- Recognizes that international partnerships are needed and aims to mobilize internal and external resources.

The World Bank initially is focusing this approach on sub-Saharan African countries with the highest HIV/AIDS prevalence rates. To this end, the World Bank has established a multisectoral AIDS Campaign Team for Africa (ACTafrica) under the offices of the African Regional Vice Presidents to stimulate and support the *Intensifying Action Against HIV/AIDS strategy*. Over time, however, the Bank's HIV/AIDS-related activities will continue and gradually be intensified in other regions with rapidly growing epidemics, including South Asia and the Caribbean. The World Bank's lending for HIV/AIDS is likely to increase as more countries turn to it for financial assistance in implementing strategies to fight the HIV/AIDS epidemic.

WHAT COULD BE DONE BY THE WORLD BANK IN THE CARIBBEAN?

The World Bank's presence in the health sector of the wider Caribbean region, except in the Dominican Republic and Haiti, is fairly small. Nevertheless, as the challenges posed by HIV/AIDS stretch well beyond the health sector alone, there is legitimate need and opportunity for World Bank partnership in the HIV/AIDS efforts in every country. As illustrated by the role it has played in AIDS and STD control projects in Brazil, Argentina and Haiti, as well as in many countries in Africa and Asia, however, the World Bank certainly has the ability to have a significant impact upon the Caribbean region's HIV/AIDS epidemic. The World Bank could expand its activities in the Caribbean both (1) by actively participating in UNAIDS and local U.N. Theme Groups on HIV/AIDS; and (2) by incorporating HIV/AIDS prevention and control activities for Caribbean countries into its country assistance programs and lending portfolios.

World Bank Participation in UNAIDS and the Local U.N. Theme Groups on HIV/AIDS

As a co-sponsor and member of UNAIDS, the World Bank has an official presence within every Caribbean nation or territory supported by UNAIDS. Thus, the World Bank might first begin its cooperation to support HIV/AIDS efforts in the Caribbean through active participation in UNAIDS and the local U.N. Theme Groups on HIV/AIDS. There are several ways in which the World Bank might act:

- First, the World Bank could provide technical support to Caribbean countries on issues such as the economic impact of HIV on the fragile economies of these countries or the process of governmental planning for HIV/AIDS within the context of evolving economic and social conditions.

- Second, the World Bank, as a UNAIDS co-sponsor, could coordinate efforts with the Inter-American Development Bank and the Caribbean Development Bank to define a lending strategy for HIV/AIDS prevention and control in the Caribbean.

- Third, the World Bank, by working with UNAIDS, could develop and strengthen ties with specific sectors—such as the finance, health, education, or tourism sectors—by providing consultative and technical support to the Caribbean regional bodies that represent Caribbean country governments and civil society.

World Bank Sector Loans and Project Support for HIV/AIDS-Related Activities in the Caribbean

The World Bank's medium-term assistance to the countries in the Caribbean, in line with the *Caribbean Regional Strategic Plan of Action for HIV/AIDS, 1999-2004,* developed with the leadership of CARICOM could parallel the World Bank's assistance in Africa:

- First, the World Bank could support efforts by the Caribbean Task Force on AIDS (see Chapter IV) to mobilize Caribbean leaders, civil society organizations, religious groups, and the private sector to intensify action against HIV/AIDS. Such support may be especially important in countries where HIV/AIDS prevalence is still low.

- Second, the World Bank could strengthen and expand its partnership with UNAIDS, the other co-sponsors of UNAIDS (UNICEF, UNDP, UNFPA, UNESCO, and PAHO/WHO), CARICOM, the Inter-American Development Bank, the Caribbean Development Bank, CAREC, the EU, NGOs, and interested bilateral agencies with a view toward implementing the *Caribbean Regional Strategic Plan of Action for HIV/AIDS, 1999-2004.*

- Finally, the World Bank could incorporate HIV/AIDS prevention and control activities for Caribbean countries in its country assistance programs and lending portfolios. The World Bank could restructure ongoing projects to finance HIV/AIDS-related activities, fund free-standing operations for the prevention and control of HIV/AIDS, and develop HIV/AIDS-related activities as part of projects in relevant non-health sectors (e.g., education, tourism). In the health sector, the World Bank could assist in strengthening the Caribbean's regional response to the HIV/AIDS epidemic as part of broader health reform efforts. As a middle-income region, much of the Caribbean currently has relatively good health care. The HIV/AIDS epidemic in the region, however, poses a threat to the fragile service delivery balance that holds these systems together. The World Bank, by participating in a multi-country dialogue—co-hosted with intergovernmental bodies such as CARICOM—could help Caribbean countries develop a stronger and more rational health care service delivery system for the Caribbean that would be better able to address needs related to HIV/AIDS. An improved health care system would at once recognize the issues pertaining to national sovereignty, address the reality that each individual nation-state cannot provide all aspects of health care delivery, and harmonize an approach consistent with the move toward the true development of a CARICOM single-market and economy. The World Bank's assistance in this realm could take many forms, including the support of individual countries to become the subregional sites for particular aspects of health care delivery.

OPERATIONALIZING AN HIV/AIDS PREVENTION AND CONTROL STRATEGY IN THE CARIBBEAN

The World Bank could finance a Multi-Country HIV/AIDS Program for the Caribbean to assist the governments of the region to scale up HIV/AIDS prevention and control activities. It would help build strong regional and national leadership with broad participation, and establish an institutional platform for long-term sustainability.

As discussed before, given the historical, social and economic factors that link the Caribbean region, as well its population movements, HIV/AIDS constitutes a regional issue. A purely "national" approach could be ineffective owing to external factors. The proposed program, therefore, would offer support to individual countries within the context of *The Caribbean Regional Strategic Plan of Action 2000-2004* prepared by the CARICOM-led Caribbean Task Force on HIV/AIDS and endorsed by the heads of Government. Additionally, by supporting a program conceived as part of regional initiative, donors can more easily exercise their preferences and comparative advantages and complement each other. This was evident at the regional HIV/AIDS Conference in September 2000, sponsored by the Government of Barbados, PAHO/WHO, UNAIDS and the World Bank. Several bilateral donors offered support to regional aspects of the Plan, while the World Bank committed resources at the country level.

In the face of the challenges posed by the HIV/AIDS epidemic, it is expected that the proposed program would support the Caribbean Governments in building political consensus, public awareness, and experience both domestically and region-wide. It would help them devote additional resources to the prevention and control of HIV/AIDS, care for persons already affected by it, experiment with institutional arrangements to curb its spread and modify them on the basis of lessons learned over time.

The program's underlying premise would be that a broad, inclusive, and in many cases experimental set of activities is needed to have a substantial impact on the spread of the epidemic, considering the diversity of sources of infection, and the behavioral and cultural factors that drive it. This means that the approach would have to be opportune, build on and scale up successes that have been achieved, and accept the costs of errant starts while learning from them.

World Bank assistance would be structured as horizontal/regional Adaptable Program Lending (APL). Under the APL, individual countries would obtain separate loans and/or credits to finance their own national HIV/AIDS Prevention and Control projects. The respective national projects would be appraised and readied for approval following provisions for investment lending. Final decision as to the countries to be included would be made based on Country Assistance Strategy (CAS) considerations and the degree of readiness of the countries.

The operational goal of the APL would be to have all the Caribbean countries participating within the next two years. Each would then seek to reach their own project objectives for HIV/AIDS prevention and control within the ensuing 5 years. The proposed APL, by visibly committing resources, to complement the activities supported by other donors, would attempt to ensure adequate resources to fund the national programs.

Structuring a Regional HIV/AIDS Program as an APL

In the Caribbean, the principal biological factors explaining this epidemic are much better understood than are the social, cultural, and economic factors that create the environment for HIV transmission. Clearly, however, the countries need to adopt and implement an operational plan for addressing the HIV/AIDS epidemic that takes all of these factors into account.

In this context of uncertainty about certain factors associated with the HIV/AIDS epidemic and how to address them, the risks of failure of an HIV/AIDS program in the Caribbean countries can be minimized by structuring a lending program that gives these countries an opportunity to build experience, political consensus, and public awareness at both within these countries and region-wide. The countries in the Caribbean need to simultaneously (1) devote resources to HIV/AIDS prevention and treatment; and (2) experiment with institutional arrangements to curb the spread of the HIV/AIDS epidemic and to treat the individuals who develop AIDS, modifying those arrangements as they learn over time.

Lastly, as in the cases of telecommunications, and disaster management programs, the multi-country program approach would simply allow the World Bank to address individual country requirements in a more cost-effective manner by maximizing the use of similarities between country situations, while respecting the fundamental differences between them. As such, in conjunction with other international organizations, the program could be designed along the lines of an existing APL—specifically, the World Bank-financed Organization of Eastern Caribbean States (OECS) Emergency Recovery and Disaster Management Recovery Program.

The first step in designing a World Bank-supported multi-country APL for HIV/AIDS prevention and control in the Caribbean countries would be to identify several "champions" who could mobilize interest and be a focal point for addressing the issues. Then, a significant dialogue among the Caribbean governments and with the donor community would be necessary to develop the APL. The following points could provide structure to such a dialogue:

- *"Letter of development program."* The basis of the World Bank's APL would be an agreed-upon statement of the program's rationale and purpose, its medium-term (5- to 10- year) goals, and the milestones that could be reached sequentially over the period. The statement would also include ways and means (including an action program, phasing, implementation, cost and financing, and monitoring and evaluation arrangements) that would be needed to reach these goals. The point of departure of such a statement would be the *Caribbean Regional Strategic Plan of Action for HIV/AIDS, 1999-2004,* formulated under CARICOM's leadership (see Chapter IV).

- *Program goals.* The APL's goals for reduced HIV/AIDS transmission and treatment in the Caribbean countries would be based solidly on the goals agreed with each country. Governments would be encouraged to establish realistic outcomes for themselves, with appropriate milestones that they could progressively reach. Depending on the lag time between an intervention and a measurable difference in the HIV/AIDS prevalence rates, it is likely that the real impacts of the program would be observable somewhat later in its implementation (a back-loaded outcome). Still, it would be useful to establish target levels for various "leading indicators" that could be monitored earlier in the program. The success of an APL would ultimately depend on the success made in developing such a hierarchy of results. For that reason, devoting a significant share of preparation resources to this effort would be warranted.

- *Common and specific activities.* There is common agreement in the Caribbean that each country could benefit from (1) the development of sustainable organizations and practices (and possibly some modification of legal and/or regulatory frameworks) to reduce HIV/AIDS transmission rates and treat people infected with HIV; (2) raising public and community awareness of HIV/AIDS and changing attitudes; and (3) improving access to resources for HIV/AIDS prevention and treatment. An APL to which each country could subscribe would contain these "components" as a minimum set. Achieving agreement on this "regional approach" would be important as part of the preparation stage of the program. Applying the framework in each "subscribing" country would then require additional local consultative processes and agreement on specifics unique to the country concerned. This activity could be considered as part of the implementation of the program, which might be complemented with provisions for financing prevention and treatment, and other activities that were justified.

- *Program phases.* The World Bank's Board of Directors agreed in the case of the OECS Emergency Recovery and Disaster Management Program to treat specific country applications of an agreed-upon regional framework as "phases" of the OECS program. A similar structure could be envisaged for a regional HIV/AIDS program in the Caribbean region:

- o Caribbean countries would be grouped according to their readiness *to undertake an initial set of activities aimed at establishing sustainable domestic structures* for preventing and treating HIV/AIDS. Some might be considered "early participants, and others "later or late." Each grouping would constitute a "phase." Given that most of Caribbean countries might be involved, it is possible that three groups or "phases" could be identified. Country activities and a modest amount of investment and operational financing would be covered by individual loan/credit agreements.

- o Some Caribbean countries might find it necessary to follow their initial efforts with a further period of project-supported institution building. The program could allow for an additional "consolidation phase" within the overall program (two such phases may be necessary, depending on the timing of progress being made by countries in the region).

- o Once a given country's institutional capacity for preventing and controlling the spread of HIV/AIDS within the country met a standard for sustainability, the country could enter a final "phase," in which it could sign loan/credit agreements allowing it access to additional funds for the support of additional investments and operations financing.

- o A region-wide consultative process in the Caribbean would help establish the country groupings.

- *Triggers and exit strategies.* The Caribbean countries would be expected to have met their own HIV/AIDS prevention and control milestones when proposing participation in new operations. Additional "triggers" for a country to advance to subsequent phases would relate to the demonstrated sustainability of their domestic HIV/AIDS management infrastructure. The World Bank would probably not wish to "exit" from this program, which is regional and in which some countries would be continuously making progress. The World Bank may, however, not follow on with new loan/credit agreements with individual countries depending on their performance and other related conditions for eligibility for World Bank financing.

- *Monitoring and evaluation (ongoing and periodic/annual).* Countries would need to develop their own monitoring and evaluation capacities to track project implementation and impact as part of their management systems. A program of this nature should also consider providing for periodic region-wide performance and results "audits" as a basis for sharing of experience.

- *Implementation and coordination arrangements.* An APL of this nature would be implemented through the collective efforts of the participating countries. However, planning for a coordination function would be important as a basis for stimulating collective learning and information sharing. An assessment of the viability of existing regional groupings to assume this function, and the incremental resources and agreements that would support the role would be necessary.

- *Cost and financing.* The level of financial support may be determined as a dialogue advances. Complementary institution-building support that might be forthcoming from bilateral and/or NGO sources should also be taken into account. At the Barbados HIV/AIDS Conference held on September 11-12, 2000, the World Bank proposed a lending package of US$100 million for HIV/AIDS activities in the region through an APL; pending approval by the Board of Directors (see Annex 1).

Coordination with the International Finance Corporation to promote private sector involvement

The International Finance Corporation (IFC) is currently working with private firms in assessing investment opportunities in the Caribbean. Building upon IFC-supported private/public partnerships (i.e., clusters), efforts could be made to enlist the participation of private firms interested in investing in the Caribbean to support HIV/AIDS prevention and control efforts as part of risk-minimization strategies (e.g., given the relative importance of tourism in the Caribbean economy, HIV/AIDS can potentially have a negative impact upon the viability of the tourism industry as a whole).

Promoting civil society participation

As it has been done in Brazil (see Box 5-2), World Bank support may help promote active involvement of civil society organizations (CSOs) in HIV/AIDS prevention and control in the Caribbean countries. To this end, a promising approach to stimulate innovative multisectoral activities might be the creation of a demand-driven fund managed by an intersectoral group headed by Ministry of Health officials and financed by public and private sources that could channel resources to public and private organizations, including community groups. Activities that could be financed by such a fund would include pilot interventions or their replication at the community level, media campaigns, and applied research on risk factor prevalence and effectiveness of interventions.

Box 5-2: Civil Society and HIV/AIDS Control in Brazil

In Brazil, the term civil society has a political connotation and refers to the vast non-governmental sector composed of community organizations, social movements, NGOs, charitable organizations, professional associations, churches and corporate foundations.

Civil society organizations (CSOs) have played a significant role in the evolution of the fight against AIDS in Brazil. The Government's response to the AIDS crisis was partly fueled by pressure from CSOs in several state capitals that were formed to support people with AIDS. These included the *GAPAs* or *Grupos de Apoio a Prevencão a AIDS*. Also, the *Associacão Brasileira Interdisciplinar de AIDS* (ABIA) brought together doctors, lawyers, sociologists, church leaders, and journalists to carry out independent research on the growing epidemic and to monitor government action. It was headed by two capable and charismatic leaders, Herbert "Betinho" de Souza and Herbert Daniel. ABIA assumed a leadership role within the AIDS civil society community.

In light of the alarming number of hemophiliacs infected through tainted blood, (85% in the city of Rio de Janeiro) ABIA mounted a successful campaign for more stringent standards in blood banks throughout the country. The lobbying campaign consisted of demonstrations in front of blood banks, letter signing campaigns, visits to the Congress, and assisting in the drafting of legislation. In 1989, an offshoot of ABIA was established in Rio de Janeiro called *Grupo Pela Vidda*. The *Pela Vidda* was comprised of HIV-positive persons and was geared toward providing care and support services to people with AIDS including legal aid, counseling, and support groups. Today these patients groups have evolved into a large national network, *Rede Nacional de Pessoas Vivendo com AIDS* (RNP+) comprised of about 400 care and support organizations.

In the late 1980s, these various organizations began to pressure the Brazilian government to take action against the epidemic. Their tactics included street demonstrations, distribution of condoms, letter writing campaigns, delegations to Brasilia to meet with the Minister of Health and the President, and distribution of flyers and other materials urging the Government to provide funding and develop AIDS prevention programs.

With time, many of the CSOs began to establish local, regional, and national AIDS/CSO networks in order to exchange information and more effectively influence public policy. Several state capital cities and regions such as Sao Paulo, Rio de Janeiro, Northeast, Centerwest, have active AIDS/CSO networks. The first national AIDS/CSO conference was held in 1989. One of the leaders of this nascent movement, Jane Galvao of ABIA, was recently appointed the head of the NC's CSO Liaison Office.

In the 1990s, the number of CSOs involved in HIV/AIDS control and prevention proliferated. Many of them were able to form as the direct result of funding made available by the Ministry of Health under a special component of the World Bank financed AIDS and STD Control Project. The 120 CSOs registered with the NC in 1992 grew over 600 today. Between 1994 and 1997, the Ministry of Health (with World Bank financing) supported 427 CSO projects costing US$ 18.1 million and involving 175 implementing organizations. The Second World Bank Aids and STD Control Project, which has been effective for about 18 months has already implemented 350 CSOs subprojects.

To date, CSO activities funded by the Ministry of Health have included research centers, social movements such as the association of transvestites, and informal community or single-constituency groups. The make-up of the organizations funded and/or their target groups have included homosexual men, feminists, transvestites, pregnant women, truck drivers, children, commercial sex workers, drug users, prisoners, hemophiliacs, and the general public.

The breadth of activities funded has included research, public education, condom distribution, patient care, policy analysis and advocacy, counseling, patient family support, organizational networking, materials production and distribution, teacher training, and networking events. CSO activities focused on behavior intervention (34%), followed by information, education and communication initiatives (31%), support to persons living with AIDS (29%), and a small number of institutional strengthening efforts (6%).

These organizations demonstrated their ability to reach groups of individuals at-risk whose needs the government was either unable or unwilling to address. The CSO projects funded over the past 8 years have distributed over a million condoms, disseminated educational materials to over half a million persons, provided specialized orientation to over 200,000 persons, and have trained over 2,000 trainers. While the impact and cost-effectiveness of CSO activities in changing high risk behaviors has yet to be quantified, CSO participation has clearly broadened the reach of control efforts into a number of key high risk, marginal and hard to reach populations.

Forging a Government/CSOs Partnership

What is most remarkable about the collaboration which has been forged between the Government and the civil society sector is that it began to become solidified at a time when overall government/CSO relations were still quite tense due to a long history of suspicion and animosity framed by the period of the military regime from 1964 to 1985. On the other hand, there were apparently several underlying reasons which led the Government to attempt an operational partnership with AIDS/CSOs.

First, the very multi-faceted and social nature of the epidemic itself. It was clear from the onset that government alone would not be able to reach the most high risk populations (IV drug users, commercial sex workers, men who have sex with men) and undertake the needed grassroots prevention and treatment work. CSOs complement government action by their flexible, innovative, and generally more cost-effective approach. Further, CSOs could reach and work effectively with people at the community level, especially with marginalized segments of society.

Second, actions which are politically difficult for the Government to undertake sometimes can be done by CSOs (harm reduction programs, for example)

Third, International development agencies such as the World Health Organization (WHO) and the World Bank clearly encouraged the NC to pursue a collaborative approach to civil society.

Source: Garrison, J., A. Abreu, and J. Sanchez Loppacher, 2000.

COST SIMULATIONS FOR HIV/AIDS PROGRAMS IN THE CARIBBEAN: MAIN ASSUMPTIONS AND RESULTS

An HIV/AIDS program cost simulation[11] for the Caribbean Region was carried out in preparation for the regional meeting on HIV/AIDS held on September 11-12, 2000, in Barbados. The purpose of the exercise was to estimate the cost of HIV/AIDS prevention and treatment packages for 23 Caribbean countries[12] under various scenarios. The model structure was loosely based on a simulation model being developed by the World Bank[13] and the parameters underlying the base scenario were obtained from the literature and from a panel of HIV/AIDS experts from PAHO, UNAIDS, the University of West Indies, and CARICOM[14].

Model Structure and Main Assumptions

The following information was collected/produced to conduct the cost simulations:

First, an exhaustive menu of prevention and treatment activities was established

An exhaustive list of the principal interventions to prevent the further transmission of the HIV virus and to mitigate the impact of HIV/AIDS on persons and communities was drawn. The list is basically a list of the typical interventions supported by HIV/AIDS programs around the world. No attempt was made to choose among these activities a priori; it was felt that the best strategy would be to prioritize these activities in a second phase (and therefore trim down the list) according to the specific financial and implementation constraints encountered on a country-by-country basis. Ideally, this would be done with additional information from a cost-effectiveness analysis that would help to rank the interventions.

A first set of "indirect" interventions includes surveillance, research, monitoring and evaluation, advocacy, and enhancing regional and national institutional capacity to carry out the programs. A second set of preventive interventions includes those activities that have strong spillover benefits to society as a whole in preventing HIV infections and thus reducing the spread of the disease. They include public awareness campaigns, programs aimed at preventing the spread from high-risk groups such as prostitutes and intravenous drug users into the general population, screening, ensuring safe blood supply, fostering behavior change, increasing access to condoms and preventing the transmission from infected mothers to their babies. The third set of interventions includes various aspects of care and financial assistance for persons or relatives of persons living with HIV/AIDS. These interventions are palliative (prevention of opportunistic infections, counseling, home-based care, anti-retroviral therapy) since there is no cure for AIDS. We also include in this set of activities support to orphans of AIDS patients.

---

11 A version of the simulation model (in Excel format) can be downloaded from:
http://wbln0018.worldbank.org/LAC/lacinfoclient.nsf/d29684951174975c85256735007fef12/ddbc64d751a7ce3185256960005de075?OpenDocument
12 The countries were loosely grouped according their geographic, cultural and economic proximity. Group 1: Anguilla, Antigua & Barbuda, British Virgin Islands, Dominica, Grenada, Montserrat, St. Kitts, St. Lucia, St. Vincent. Group 2: Bahamas, Bermuda, Cayman, Turks & Caicos. Group 3: Haiti, Dominican Republic. Group 4: Netherlands Antilles, Aruba, Guyana, Suriname. Group 5: Barbados, Belize, Jamaica, Trinidad & Tobago. Group 6: Cuba
13 Bonnel R., et al., 'The Cost of Scaling-Up HIV/AIDS Programs to a National Level for Sub-Saharan Africa,' Working Paper, World Bank, April 2000.
14 The team of experts collegially decided upon parameter values during a two-day workshop held in Trinidad and Tobago (August 17 – 18, 2000).

Unit costs were then assigned to each activity

Unit costs were then estimated for each of these activities. The costs were for the most part taken from the simulation exercise that is being undertaken in Sub-Saharan Africa[15]. The information derives from the literature and from the direct experience of the team of experts with HIV/AIDS programs in developing world settings. These costs should be revised as Caribbean-specific data become available. Some of the costs are expressed as a the sum of a fixed and of a variable component. The fixed component represents the cost below which the intervention cannot be conducted meaningfully, while the variable component (expressed as a multiplier of per capita public spending in health) is an implicit recognition of the budget constraints affecting each country[16].

Table 5-1: Illustrative Annual Cost Assumptions

Intervention	Cost per...	Low Cost Scenario	High Cost Scenario
Overhead Activities	Capita	$0.10 - $0.50	$0.10 - $0.50
Surveillance	Capita	$1	$2
Targeted Interventions for Commercial Sex Workers (CSW)	CSW	$16	$21
Syndromic Management of Sexually Transmitted Infections (STI)	Case	$13	$16
Treatment of Opportunistic Infections	Case	$210 + three times public spending	$2,100
Home-based Care	Case	$500	$1,200
Anti-Retroviral Therapy (HAART)	Case	$7,000	$10,000

Source: World Bank/University of West Indies/CAREC/UNAIDS/PAHO/WHO estimates

The relevant population and epidemiological information was compiled

Estimates for the model parameters were collected or extrapolated from the latest published sources or generated by the panel of experts who participated in the simulation exercise. The main variables used by the model are: population, HIV prevalence, birth rates, access to health services, use of ante-natal care services, ante-natal care HIV prevalence, percentage of sexually active population reporting non-regular partnerships, annual incidence of treatable sexually transmitted infections (STIs), proportion of STIs that are symptomatic, average annual number of commercial sex acts/sex worker, prevalence of syphilis among women, cumulative number of orphans, HIV prevalence rates among high-risk groups (prisoners, men who have sex with men, commercial sex workers, military), migrant and tourist populations, and public spending per capita in health.

Finally, program coverage assumptions were constructed

The final set of model inputs were the coverage assumptions. For nearly all the interventions contemplated, it was assumed that 100 percent of the relevant population was targeted (e.g., all commercial sex workers, all HIV-infected mothers, all youngsters in school, etc). There were two main departures from the universal coverage assumption: it was assumed that only 20 percent of AIDS patients would benefit from home-based care, and that only 50

---

15 See footnote 2.
16 This contradicts, at the margin, the earlier claim that budget constraints are factored only later in the simulation exercise. This peculiar way of expressing certain costs parameters is no more than an attempt to compromise between divergent expert opinions.

percent of HIV patients would benefit from highly active antiretroviral therapy (HAART), the three- and four-drug combinations against HIV. A 100-percent coverage was deemed improbable for these two interventions if only because the health system cannot reach all patients and because the take up of home-based care is partly predicated on client behavior. The cost estimates derived from the model are shown to be extremely sensitive to the coverage assumptions.

Main Results

Using the assumptions detailed in the previous section, the following results were derived:

Table 5-2: Low Cost Package

Program	Total Cost with HAART (US$ million)	Percent of Total	Total Cost w/o HAART (US$ million)	Percent of Total
"Indirect activities"	51.1	2%	51.1	9%
Public Awareness and Prevention	162.1	5%	162.1	28%
Basic Care	362.2	11%	362.2	63%
HAART	2,760.4	83%	0.0	0%
Total	3,335.8	100%	575.4	100%

Source: World Bank/University of West Indies/CAREC/UNAIDS/PAHO/WHO estimates

The cost of providing a comprehensive package of prevention and care activities for 100 percent of the relevant population the Caribbean would therefore be prohibitively expensive. Table 3 below shows how these costs would translate into per capita terms for a few countries and compares the estimated HIV/AIDS program costs with current overall per capita spending on health.

Table 5-3: Per Capita Costs (US$)

Country	Per capita health spending	Preventive Program	Plus Basic Care Program	Plus HAART
Bahamas	$785	$8	$69	$220
Haiti	$18	$6	$18	$206
Dominican Republic	$91	$4	$15	$117
Guyana	$45	$6	$22	$204
Jamaica	$149	$4	$15	$89
Trinidad and Tobago	$197	$4	$16	$91

Source: World Bank/University of West Indies/CAREC/UNAIDS/PAHO/WHO estimates

Launching a comprehensive package of interventions (prevention, basic care, HAART) would bump up the current overall spending in health from 28 percent in the Bahamas, all the way to more than a 1,000 percent in Haiti. However, the spread of the disease can probably be reversed through preventive programs with the addition of some of the highest priority basic care activities, and these interventions are feasible everywhere. The HAART costs are probably overstated because efforts are being made to reduce the cost of retroviral drugs. Nevertheless, as the price of the treatment falls, its use may expand sufficiently to keep total expenditures on HAART quite high.

Policy Implications

The programs can clearly not be applied in toto or to the same degree in each country. In a follow-up analysis, the University of West Indies modified some of the parameters to better reflect budget constraints and the limited implementation capacity of Caribbean countries (especially Haiti) to come up with much smaller cost estimates ($258 million in the low unit cost scenario).

The cost simulation instrument that was developed is best used at country-level. First, policymakers can correct the assumptions as needed, and use population, epidemiological, cost and coverage parameters that are closer to reality. Second, policymakers have a better sense of the budget and implementation constraints the country faces and can tailor the programs accordingly. Since countries in the Caribbean Region will necessarily have to choose from the menu of options because they simply cannot afford all of them, priority-setting is of crucial importance. It is important that the criteria for choosing among options be clear and explicit and aim to achieve maximum impact in terms of reduction of the transmission of the virus and in terms of reducing the impact of HIV/AIDS on persons and families[17].

Conclusion

No single step will suffice to curb the relentless spread of the HIV/AIDS epidemic in the countries of the Caribbean. What is needed is a balanced combination of advocacy, incentives, disincentives, funding, and policy support. The overarching goal of support for developing countries from the World Bank and other development partners should be to help every country at risk to establish an appropriate national HIV/AIDS program comprising basic prevention, basic treatment, and basic care. It should be clear, however, that while costly drugs are available to a small percentage of the world's people, behavior change is the only way to safeguard against infection in most of the world. Concerted action by Caribbean governments and Caribbean regional agencies such as the CARICOM, in partnership with civil society, the private sector and NGOs, and with the assistance of the international community, will help to mitigate the adverse impact of AIDS on people of the Caribbean region in years to come.

---

17 Such an exercise was successfully conducted in the Dominican Republic at the end of September 2000 as part of the preparation for a World Bank-financed project. The main criterion that was used to prioritize among activities was expected cost-effectiveness.

ANNEX 1

CARIBBEAN CONFERENCE ON HIV/AIDS
BARBADOS, 11 AND 12 SEPTEMBER 2000, SUMMARY STATEMENT

The Caribbean Conference on HIV/AIDS, sponsored by the Government of Barbados together with the CARICOM Secretariat, PAHO/WHO, UNAIDS and the World Bank took place in Barbados on 11 and 12 September 2000. Participants included governments from the English, Spanish, French and Dutch speaking countries and territories, representatives of Caribbean regional organizations, UN agencies, multilateral and bilateral agencies, civil society and associations of people living with HIV/AIDS, academic institutions and the media. Present at the Conference were Prime Ministers of Barbados, the Bahamas, St Vincent and the Grenadines and St Kitts and Navis, the Chief Minister of Anguilla, as well as ministers of health, population and/or social development from The Bahamas (also represented by the Minister of Finance), Barbados (represented by cabinet), Belize, Cuba, Dominica, Grenada, Haiti, Jamaica, St Kitts and Nevis, St Lucia, Trinidad and Tobago, Turks and Caicos, representatives of the Presidential Commission on AIDS from the Dominican Republic as well as high level representatives from Antigua & Barbuda, Aruba, Guyana, Montserrat and Suriname. The meeting was organized following a decision of the Caribbean Group on Cooperation in Economic Development (CGCED) which met in June 2000 in Washington, D.C.

THE MEETING RECOGNIZED

- The gravity of the HIV/AIDS situation in the region. The Caribbean is the hardest-hit region in the world outside sub-Saharan Africa.
- Out of the 12 countries with the highest HIV prevalence in the Americas 9 are in the Caribbean.
- AIDS is already the leading cause of death among men and women in the 15 to 44 age group.
- The epidemic continues to spread and has a devastating social and economic impact.
- Intolerance, homophobia and discrimination of people living with HIV/AIDS and of those vulnerable to infection drive the epidemic underground and contribute to the further spread of the virus.
- HIV/AIDS is increasingly recognized as a major development problem throughout the Caribbean.
- Investing in HIV/AIDS now will significantly reduce future costs. A conservative estimate of the cost of a comprehensive response to the epidemic in the Caribbean would be in the order of US$ 260 million per year. This is more than a ten-fold increase compared to the level of current national and international spending in the Caribbean per year.

- Mobilizing the required funding will require creative solutions and an increased commitment at national level from governments and the private sector as well as support by the international community.

The meeting endorsed the regional strategic Plan developed by the Caribbean Task Force on HIV/AIDS as the framework on which to base an expanded response to the epidemic. To be effective, this response has to be pan-Caribbean in scope.

THE MEETING CONCLUDED THAT

- Leadership at the highest political level is essential to the response.

- Given its developmental impact, HIV/AIDS needs to be addressed through a multi-sectoral approach.

- To move forward it is necessary to reduce stigma, discrimination and exclusion of people living with and affected by HIV/AIDS and protect their human rights and dignity.
- People living with HIV/AIDS should be supported and integrated fully into the national responses to the epidemic.

- Prevention efforts must be strengthened and broadened.

- Increased access to quality care and treatment is needed now.

- Strengthening the management and operational capacity of national AIDS programs is essential to ensure an effective and sustainable response.

- The private sector should be encouraged to become an active partner in the response.

- Reinforcing positive social and cultural norms and values as well as healthy behaviors is an important part of the response.

SUPPORT FOR THE REGIONAL RESPONSE

- The meeting represented a commitment of the participating Caribbean Governments to increase the levels of resources, both human and financial, that will be made available to address the epidemic in their countries.

- Proposals for more involvement of the private sector, e.g. through the creation of a Caribbean Business Council on HIV/AIDS were also discussed.

- The international community pledged to support intensified action in the Caribbean with both financial and technical assistance.

- Pledges of continued and/or increased support were made by the governments of The Netherlands, Canada, USA, Germany, United Kingdom and France, as well as by the UN system and multilateral agencies (including the European Commission, the Caribbean Development Bank and the Inter-American Development Bank).

- The World Bank proposed a lending package of US$ 85 to 100 million for HIV/AIDS activities in the countries of the region (pending approval by their Board).

- It is expected that additional financial commitments will be made by all partners both for the Regional Plan of Action as well as for national level efforts.

NEXT STEPS

- Establish an International Partnership on HIV/AIDS in the Caribbean building upon existing processes and structures.
- Develop an operational plan for implementing the Regional Strategy including the definition of institutional arrangements.
- Establish clear links between the Regional Strategic Plan and national level action.

Journal Articles and Publications

Ainsworth, M., L, Fransen, and M. Over, eds. 1998. *Confronting AIDS: Evidence from the Developing World.* European Commission/World Bank. Luxembourg: Office for Publications of the European Communities.

Ahlburg, A., and ER Jensen. 1998. "The Economics of the Commercial Sex Industry." In: M. Ainsworth, L. Fransen, and M. Over, eds. *Confronting AIDS: Evidence from the Developing World.* European Commission/World Bank. Luxembourg:Office for Publications of the European Communities.

Adu-Krow, W., R. Barber-Madden, Z. Stein. 1989. MCH Program, et al. International Conference of AIDS. Jun 4-9;5:911.

Baldwin, K. 1999. "HIV/AIDS in the Caribbean." *Caribbean Health* 2(1):23-24.

Becker, J., and E. Kirberger. 1997. "A Sexual and Reproductive Health Approach in Latin America and the Caribbean (letter to the editor)." *American Journal of Public Health* 87:692-693.

Behets, F., A. Brathwaite, L. Bennet, et al. 1997. "The Decentralization of Syphilis Screening for Prompt Treatment and Improved Contact Tracing in Jamaican Public Clinics." Collaborative Working Group on Decentralized Syphilis Screening. *American Journal of Public Health* 87(6):1019-1021.

Behets, F., E. Genece, M. Narcisse, et al. 1998. "Approaches to Control Sexually Transmitted Diseases in Haiti," 1992-95. *Bulletin of the World Health Organization* 76(2):189-194.

Black, B. 1996. "Cross-Fertilization: HIV/AIDS Prevention Strategies Cross Borders. *AIDScaptions*, 3(3):19-23.

Bonnel, R., et al. 2000. "The Cost of Scaling-Up HIV/AIDS Programs to a National Level for Sub-Saharan Africa." Working Paper, World Bank.

Brathwaite, AR., JP. Figueroa, and E. Ward. 1997. "A Comparison of Prevalence Rates of Genital Ulcers among Persons Attending a Sexually Transmitted Disease Clinic in Jamaica." *West Indian Medical Journal*, 46(3):67-71.

Cáceres, Uraña. 1998. *La Mortalidad Materna en la República Dominicana.* Santo Domingo: UNFPA.

Camara, B., N. Shelton, and R. McLean. 1997. "Modeling and Projecting HIV and Its Economic Impact in the Caribbean: The Experience of Trinidad and Tobago and Jamaica" (working paper).

Camara, B., et al. 1998. *HIV/AIDS Situation.* Report—UNECTG meeting.

Camara, B., HU Wagner, CJ. Hopedales, et al. 1998. "Evaluation of STD/HIV/AIDS surveillance systems in five Caribbean countries." *12th World AIDS Conference,* Geneva, June 28th-July 3rd, 1998 (Abstract 43451).

Caribbean Task Force on HIV/AIDS. 2000a. *HIV/AIDS in the Caribbean: Addressing the Challenges and Opportunities for Strengthening the National and Regional Response to the Epidemic.* Prepared with the support of UNAIDS. June 2000.

——— 2000b. *The Caribbean Regional Strategic Plan for HIV/AIDS 1999-2004.* February 2000.

Castro, L., and Y. Espino. 1992. "Impact of Gay Organization Practice on AIDS Preventive Behavior in a Homophobic Society." 8th International Conference on AIDS/III STD World Congress, Amsterdam, The Netherlands (Poster PoD-5177).

Celentano, DD., KE. Nelson, C. Beyrer, et al. 1998. "Decreasing Incidence of HIV and Sexually Transmitted Diseases in Young Thai Men: Evidence for Success of the HIV/AIDS Control and Prevention Program. *AIDS*" 12(5):F29-36.

Centers for Disease Control and Prevention (CDC). 1998. Administration of Zidovudine During Pregnancy and Delivery to Prevent Perinatal HIV Tansmission—Thailand, 1996-1998. *Morbidity and Mortality Weekly Report (MMWR)* 47(8):151-154.

——— 1999a *Compendium of HIV Prevention Interventions with Evidence of Effectiveness.* CDC's HIV/AIDS Prevention Research Synthesis Project. Atlanta.

——— 1999b. "Global Burden of Tuberculosis. Estimated Incidence, Prevalence, and Mortality by Country." *Journal of the American Medical Association* 282(7):677-686.

——— 1999c. Increases in Unsafe Sex and Rectal Gonorrhea among Men who Have Sex with Men—San Francisco, 1994-1997. *Morbidity and Mortality Weekly Report (MMWR)* 48:45-8.

Chun, T-W., D. Engel, SB Mizell, et al. 1999. "Effect of Interleukin-2 on the Pool of Latently Infected, Resting CD4 T Cells in HIV-1 Infected Patients Receiving Highly Active Anti-retroviral Therapy." *Nature Medicine* 5(6):651.

Coates, T., G. Coates, G. Sangiwa G, et al. 1998. "Serodiscordant Married Couples Undergoing Couples Counseling and Testing Reduce Risk Behavior with each other but not with Extra-Marital Partners." *12th World AIDS Conference,* Geneva, June 28th-July 3rd, 1998 (Abstract 33268).

Coates, T., G. Sangiwa, D. Balmer, et al. 1998. "Voluntary HIV Counseling and Testing (VCT) Reduces Risk Behavior in Developing Countries: Results from the Voluntary Counseling and Testing Study." *12th World AIDS Conference,* Geneva, June 28th-July 3rd, 1998 (Abstract 33269).

Cuchi, P., and D. Patz. 1998. "Mosaic of the AIDS epidemics in Latin America and the Caribbean." *Journal of the International Association of Physicians in AIDS Care* 4(7):36-7.

Cuchi, P., M. Weissenbacher, G. Schumunis, et al. 1998. "Ensuring Blood Safety in Latin America and the Caribbean (LAC): A Cost-Effective Strategy." *12th World AIDS Conference,* Geneva, June 28th-July 3rd, 1998 (Abstract 33204).

Cuchi, P., B. Schwartlander, K. Stanecki, et al. 1998. "HIV/AIDS/STD epidemiological fact sheets: a new tool for surveillance in Latin America and the Caribbean (LAC)." *12th World AIDS Conference,* Geneva, June 28th-July 3rd, 1998 (Abstract 60641).

Dadian, MJ. 1997. "Condom Sales Boom as Rwanda and Haiti Struggle to Rebuild." *AIDScaptions,* 4(1):4-9.

Dadian, MJ. 1998. "Improving Access to Antiretroviral Therapy in Latin America. *Impact on HIV.*" online (www.fhi.org), 1(1).

De Grouland, M., U. Wagner, and B. Camara. 1998. "Analysis of the Situation of HIV/AIDS in the English-speaking Caribbean." *12th World AIDS Conference,* Geneva, June 28th-July 3rd, 1998 (Abstract 13164).

De Moya, EA., R. Garcia, Instituto de Sexualidad Humana/OASD, Santo Domingo, Republica Dominicana. "A 'gay paradise' revisited: perceived HIV/AIDS impact on the male sex industry in Santo Domingo." Int. Conf AIDS. 1998;12:977 (abstract no. 44205).

Du Boisrouvray, A. 2000. "The Global Impact of AIDS." Speech given at the World Bank, Washington, DC, Jan. 24, 2000.

Eggleston, E., J. Jackson, and K. Hardee. 1999. "Sexual Attitudes and Behavior among Young Adolescents in Jamaica." *International Family Planning Perspectives* 25(2):78-84.

European Union (EU). 1999. "Strengthening the Institutional Response to HIV/AIDS in the Caribbean" Project Proposal. Working Document.

Field, and Dallabetta. 1997. "Integrated reproductive health services: where do we go from here?" *AIDScaptions* 4(1):40-43.

Figueroa, JP., and AR. Brathwaite. 1995. "Is under-reporting of AIDS a problem in Jamaica?" *West Indian Medical Journa,* 44:51-54.

Figueroa, JP., A. Brathwaite, E. Ward, et al. 1995. "The HIV/AIDS Epidemic in Jamaica." *AIDS* 9(7):761-8.

Figueroa, JP., AR. Brathwaite, M. Wedderburn, et al. 1998. "Is HIV/STD control in Jamaica making a difference?" *AIDS* 12 Suppl 2:S89-98.

Furtado, M., DS. Callaway, JP. Phair, et al. 1999. "Persistence of HIV-1 Transcription in Peripheral-Blood Mononuclear Cells in Patients Receiving Potent Antiretroviral Therapy." *New England Journal of Medicine* 340(21):1614-22.

Forsythe, S. 1998. "The Affordability of Antiretroviral Therapy in Developing Countries: What Policymakers Need to Know. *AIDS* 12 Suppl 2: S11-8.

Forsythe, S., and C. Gilks. 1998. "Policymaking and ARVs: a Framework for Rational Decision Making (opinion)." *Impact on HIV* online (www.fhi.org), 1(1).

Forsythe, S., and C. Gilks. 1999. "Economic Issues and Antiretroviral Therapy in Developing Countries." *Trans Royal Society of Tropical Medicine and Hygiene,* Jan-Feb 93(1):1-3.

Forsythe, S., J. Hasbun, and M. Butler de Lister. 1998. "Protecting paradise: tourism and AIDS in the Dominican Republic." *Health Policy Planning,* 13(3):277-86.

Forsythe, S., and B. Rau. 1998. "Evolution of socioeconomic impact assessments of HIV/AIDS." *AIDS* 12 Suppl. 2:S47-55.

Forsythe, S., E. Schvartz, B. Janowitz, et al. 1992. "Measuring Costs and Benefits of Targeted Condom Distribution Programs in Latin American and Caribbean Countries." *8th International Conference on AIDS/III STD World Congress,* Amsterdam, The Netherlands (Poster PoD-5403).

Fowler, MG., J. Bertolli, and P. Nieburg. 1999. "When is Breast-Feeding not Best? the Dilemma Facing HIV-Infected Women in Resource-poor Settings." *Journal of the American Medical Association* 282(8):781-783.

Fox, LJ., NE. Williamson, W. Cates, Jr., et al. 1995. "Improving Reproductive Health: Integrating STD and Contraceptive Services." *Journal of the American Medical Women Association* 50(3-4):129-36.

Gardner, R., et al. 1999. *Closing the Gap.* Population Reports. Series H, No. 9. Baltimore, MD: Johns Hopkins University School of Public Health, Population Information Program. April 1999.

Garrison, J., A. Abreu, and J. Sanchez Loppacher. 2000. Government and civil society in the fight against HIV and AIDS in Brazil. Presented at *The Challenge of Health Reform: Reaching the Poor. Europe and the Americas Forum on Health Sector Reform,* San Jose, Costa Rica, May 24-26, 2000.

Gebo, KA., RE. Chaisson, JG. Folkemer, et al. 1999. Costs of HIV Medical Care in the Era of Highly Active Antiretroviral Therapy. *AIDS* 13:963-969.

Gomez, M., et al. 1993. Antibiotic-resistant *M. Tuberculosis* in HIV Infected and Noninfected Patients in the Bahamas. *7th World AIDS Conference* (Abstract PO-B07-1217).

Gregorich, S., et al. 1998. "Sexual Risk Behavior, Knowledge, and Attitudes in a Population-Based Probability Sample of North and Central Trinidad, West Indies: Results from the Voluntary HIV Counseling and Testing Study (VHCTS)." *12th World AIDS Conference,* Geneva, June 28th-July 3rd, 1998 (Abstract 13165).

Gwatkin, DR., and M. Guillot. 2000. *The Burden of Disease Among The Global Poor: Current Situation, Future Trends, and Implications for Strategy.* Washington, DC: World Bank.

Helquist, M., et al. 1992. Policy and Controversy in Condom Marketing Campaigns. *8th International Conference on AIDS/III STD World Congress,* Amsterdam, The Netherlands (Poster PoD-5545).

Henry, K. 1997. "Jamaicans Begin to Embrace Safer Sex." *AIDScaptions,* 4(1):18-22.

Henry, K. 1998. "Study Shows Voluntary Counseling and Testing Promotes HIV Prevention." *Impact on HIV* online (www.fhi.org), 1(1).

Hogg, RS., et al. 1998. "One World, One Hope: the Cost of Providing Antiretroviral Therapy to all Nations." *AIDS* 12:2203-2209.

Inter-American Development Bank, Pan American Health Organization/World Health Organization. 1997. *Caribbean Regional Health Study.* Washington, DC.

Izazola-Licea, JA., ed. 1996. "AIDS: The State of the Art." A review based on the *11th International Conference on AIDS* in Vancouver. Mexico, D.F.: FUSALUD/SIDALAC.

Izazola-Licea, JA., et al., ed. 1998. "Situacion Epidemiologica y Economica del SIDA en America Latina y el Caribe." Mexico, D.F.: FUSALUD/SIDALAC.

Johns Hopkins AIDS Service online (http://www.hopkins-aids.edu).

Kalichman, SC., B. Ramachandran, and S. Catz. 1999. "Adherence to Combination Antiretroviral Therapies in HIV Patients of Low Health Literacy." *Journal of General Internal Medicine* 14(5):267-73.

Katabira, E., F. Mubiru, and E. Van Praag. 1998. "Care for People Living with HIV/AIDS." *World Health* 51(6):16-17.

Lamptey, P., and W. Cates. 1996. "An ounce of Prevention is Worth a Million Lives (opinion)," *AIDScaptions* 3(3):33-35.

Levi, J. 1998. "Anonymous HIV Testing and Medical Care (letter)." *Journal of the American Medical Association* 281:2282.

Ley sobre el Sindrome de Inmunodeficiencia Adquirida (SIDA) (Ley No. 5593, 31 de Diciembre de 1993). In: V. Suero, "Leyes Sobre Salud de la Republica Dominicana," pp. 135-142.

MAP (Monitoring the AIDS Epidemic). 1998. *The Status and Trends of the HIV/AIDS Epidemics in the World: Final Report.* Veyrier du Lac, France.

MacNeil, J. 1998. Preventing Mother-to-child Transmission of HIV. Impact on HIV online (www.fhi.org), 1(1).

Marshall, D. 1998. "HIV/AIDS and Patterns of Mobility in the Caribbean: Policies and Strategic Priorities for Interventions." Caribbean Consultation on HIV/AIDS: Strategies and Resources for a Co-ordinated Regional Response.

McCarthy M. 1997. "Developing Nations Need to Integrate STD Care." *Lancet* 349(9063):1454.

McEvoy, M., 2000. "Status of the HIV/AIDS Epidemic in the Caribbean Region." Presented at Conference Heightening Awareness of HIV/AIDS in the Caribbean Region: Bridging the Gap from Denial to Acceptance to Prevention: Preparing for the Next Millennium.

McGregor, J. 1999. Presented at the Annual Clinical Meeting of the American College of Obstetricians and Gynecologists, Philadelphia.

Miotti, PG., ET. Taha, NI. Kumwenda, et al. 1999. "HIV Transmission Through Breast-feeding: A Study in Malawi." *Journal of the American Medical Association* 282(8):744-749.

Montaner, JS., V. Montessori, R. Harrigan, et al. 1999. Antiretroviral therapy: "the state of the art" (review). *Biomedical Pharmacotherapy* 53(2)63-72.

Nathanson, N., and J. Auerbach. 1999. Confronting the HIV Pandemic (editorial). *Science* 284(4):1619.

Newton, EAC., FMM. White, DC. Sokal, et al. 1994. "Modeling the HIV/AIDS Epidemic in the English-speaking Caribbean." *Bulletin of the Pan American Health Organization* 28:239-249.

News. 1999. *Caribbean Health* 2(1):4-5.

Pan American Health Organization/World Health Organization. 1997. *Health Conditions in the Caribbean.* Washington, DC.

Pan American Health Organization/World Health Organization, 1998. *Health Conditions in the Americas.* Vols. 1 and 2. Washington, DC.

Pan American Health Organization/World Health Organization. 2000. *AIDS Surveillance in the Americas. Biannual report.* February, 2000. Washington, DC.

Pan American Health Organization/World Health Organization. 2000. *Tuberculosis Control in the Americas: Country Profiles, 2000.* Washington, DC.

Pomerantz, R. 1999. "Residual HIV-1 Disease in the Era of Highly Active Antiretroviral Therapy." *New England Journal of Medicine* 340(21):1672-74.

Q&A. 1996. "Condom Social Marketing Boosts Entire Condom Market in Brazil." *AIDScaptions* 3(3):36-38.

Research for Sex Work. 1998. Amsterdam, The Netherlands: Health Care and Culture, Medical Faculty, Vrije Universiteit, June 1998 (p. 10).

Roach, TC., et al. 1996. "Clinical Management Guidelines of HIV/AIDS in Adults and Children in the Caribbean." *10th World AIDS Conference* (Abstract Th.B.4127).

Roach, TC., and EC. Hall. 1998. "Carnival AIDS," AIDS education utilizing carnival street bands. *12th World AIDS Conference,* Geneva, June 28th-July 3rd, 1998 (Abstract 43182).

Royal Tropical Institute (KIT) and Southern Africa AIDS Information Dissemination Service (SAFAIDS). *Facing the Challenges of HIV/AIDS/STDs: A Gender-Based Response*, 1998 (3rd edition).

Scott, P., and J. Becker. 1995. "HIV Prevention and Family Planning: Integration Improves Client Services in Jamaica." *AIDScaptiosn* 2(3):15-18.

Shapiro, M., et al. 1999. "Variations in the Care of HIV-infected Adults in the United States: Results from the HIV Cost and Services Utilization Study." *Journal of the American Medical Association* 281(24):2305-2315.

Stecklov, G. 1999. "Fertility Implications of Reduced Breast-feeding by HIV/AIDS-infected Mothers in Developing Countries." *American Journal of Public Health* 89(5):780.

Stephenson, J. 1997. "Health Agencies Update: Reproductive Health." *Journal of the American Medical Association* 277(24):1924.

Stiglitz, JE. 1999. "Incentives and Institutions in the Provision of Health Care in Developing Countries: Toward an Efficient and Equitable Health Care Strategy." Presented to the International Health Economics Association Meetings, Rotterdam, The Netherlands, June 7, 1999.

Tabet, SR., EA. de Moya, KK. Holmes, et al. 1996. "Sexual Behaviors and Risk Factors for HIV Infection among Men who Have Sex with Men in the Dominican Republic." *AIDS* 10(3):201-6.

Taylor, N., A. Haddix, and M. Huggins. 1996. "Cost Analysis: HIV/AIDS in the Workplace—Educational Seminars in the Caribbean Island of St. Kitts." *10th World AIDS Conference* (Abstract Mo.D.1846).

Toffolon-Weiss, M., JT. Bertrand, and SS. Terrell. 1999. "The Results Framework: an Innovative Tool for Program Planning and Evaluation." *Evaluation Review* 23(3):336-359.

UK NGO AIDS Consortium Working Group on Access to Treatment for HIV in Developing Countries. 1998. Access to Treatment for HIV in Developing Countries; Statement from International Seminar on Access to Treatment for HIV in Developing Countries, London, June 5 and 6, 1998. *Lancet* 352(9137):1379-80, 1998.

UNAIDS. 1997. *Tuberculosis and AIDS*. Best Practice Collection—Point of View. Geneva.

UNAIDS. 1998. *HIV-Related Opportunistic Diseases*. Best Practice Collection—Technical Updates. Geneva.

UNAIDS. 1998. *NGO Perspectives on Access to HIV-Related Drugs in 13 Latin American and Caribbean Countries*. Geneva.

UNAIDS. 1998. *Report on the Global HIV/AIDS Epidemic*. Geneva: World Health Organization, June.

UNAIDS. 1998. *Social Marketing: An Effective Tool in the Global Response to HIV/AIDS.* Geneva.

UNAIDS. 1999. *The Action Brief.* Issue 7, June/July 1999.

UNAIDS. 1999. *AIDS Epidemic Update.* Geneva: UNAIDS/WHO, December.

UNAIDS. 1999. *Comfort and Hope: Six Case Studies on Mobilizing Family and Community Care for and by People with HIV/AIDS.* Best Practice Collection—Case Studies. Geneva.

UNAIDS. 1999. *HIV/AIDS Prevention in the Context of New Therapies.* Best Practice Collection—Key Materials. Geneva: June 1999.

UNAIDS. 1999. *LISTEN, LEARN, LIVE! 1999 World AIDS Campaign: Challenges for Latin America and the Caribbean.* Brasilia, Feb. 25, 1999.

UNAIDS. 1999. *Summary Booklet of Best Practices (Issue 1).* Best Practice Collection—Key Materials. Geneva: June 1999.

UNAIDS. 1999. *Trends in HIV Incidence and Prevalence: Natural Course of the Epidemic or Results of Behavioral Change?* Geneva.

UNAIDS. 1999. *UNAIDS and Nongovernmental Organizations.* Best Practice Collection—Key Materials. Geneva: June 1999.

UNAIDS. 1999. *The UNAIDS Report.* Geneva: June 1999.

UNAIDS/The Francois-Xavier Bagnoud Center. 1999. *Level and Flow of National and International Resources for the Response to HIV/AIDS, 1996-1997.* Geneva.

UNAIDS/WHO. 2000. *Guidelines for Second Generation HIV Surveillance.* Geneva.

UNAIDS, WHO, and UNICEF. 1998. *Consensus Statement on Infant Feeding and HIV.* Geneva: WHO.

UNDP. *Various years.* Human Development Report. New York: Oxford University Press.

UNICEF. 1999. *The State of the World's Children.* New York.

U.S. Public Health Service/Infectious Diseases Society of America. 1999. Guidelines for the prevention of opportunistic infections in persons infected with human immunodeficiency virus. *Morbidity and Mortality Recommendations and Reports.* Vol. 48, No. RR-10.

Werker, D., S. Blount, and FM. White. 1994. "The Control of Tuberculosis in the Caribbean." *West Indian Medical Journal* 43(2):48-51.

Wheeler, V., and K. Radcliffe. 1994. "HIV infection in the Caribbean." *International Journal of STD and AIDS* 5:79-89.

Winsbury R. 1999. "HIV Vaccine Development: Would more (public) Money Bring quicker Results? *AIDS Analysis Africa* 10 (1):11-13.

Wint, B. 1999. "HIV/AIDS and Implications for the Labor Sector in the Caribbean." Presented at the Labor Ministers of the Caribbean Meeting. April 27-28, 2000, Kingston, Jamaica.

World Bank. 1993. *World Development Report 1993: Investing in Health.* Oxford and elsewhere: Oxford University Press.

World Bank. 1997. *Jamaica. Violence and Urban Poverty in Jamaica: Breaking the Cycle.* Report No. 15895-JM. Jan. 31.

World Bank. 1997. *Project Appraisal Document for the Dominican Republic Provincial Health Services Project.* Report No. 17199-DO.

World Bank. 1998. *Confronting AIDS: Public Priorities in a Global Epidemic.* New York: Oxford University Press.

Work Bank. 1999. *Responding to the Crisis: The Intensified Action Against HIV/AIDS in Africa.* Draft strategic plan. Washington, DC: March 1999.

World Bank. 2000a. *Caribbean Education Sector Strategy 2020.* Washington, DC.

——— 2000b. *Intensifying Action Against HIV/AIDS.* World Bank Development Committee, Apr. 17, 2000. SecM2000-85.

WHO (World Health Organization). 1999. *Removing Obstacles to Healthy Development. Report on Infectious Diseases.* Geneva.

Wolfensohn, JD. 2000a. Challenges facing the Bank in the 21st century. Remarks at the National Press Club, Washington, DC, Mar. 14, 2000.

——— 2000b. Free from poverty, free from AIDS. First appearance by World Bank President before the UN Security Council. New York, Jan. 10, 2000.

——— 2000c. Rethinking development—challenges and opportunities. Remarks at the Tenth Ministerial Meeting of the UN Conference on Trade and Development, Bangkok, Thailand, Feb. 16, 2000.

Zacarias, F., ML. Garcia, JL. Valdespino Gomez, et al. 1994. "HIV/AIDS and its Interaction with Tuberculosis in Latin America and the Caribbean. *Bulletin of the Pan American Health Organization* 28(4):312-23.

Zacarias, F., et al. 1998. "Glimmers of Hope: Selected STD Control Approaches in Latin America and the Caribbean." *12th World AIDS Conference,* Geneva, June 28th-July 3rd, 1998 (Abstract 43528).

Zhang, L., B. Ramratnam, K. Tenner-Racz, et al. 1999. "Quantifying Residual HIV-1 Replication in Patients Receiving Combination Antiretroviral therapy." *New England Journal of Medicine* 340(21):1605-13.

Media Articles and Wire Reports

Altman, LK. 1999. "In Africa, a Deadly Silence about Aids is Lifting. *The New York Times*. July 13, 1999 (p. D7).

Assavanonda, A. 1999. "Cheaper Treatment for HIV likely to be Cleared for Sale Soon. *Bangkok Post* online. June 8, 1999.

The Associated Press (AP). 1999. "AIDS to cost Trinidad and Tobago 4.2% Of GDP in 2000– Study." Apr. 5, 1999.

Bernstein, N. 1999. "For Subjects in Haiti Study, Free AIDS Care has a Price." *New York Times*. June 6, 1999 (p. 1, Sect. 1).

Best, R. 1999. "AIDS Figures still Mounting." *Barbados Nation* online. Mar. 9, 1999.

Brown, D. 1999. "A Low-cost Way to Cut Mother-to-child HIV?" *The Washington Post*. July 15, 1999 (p. A04).

Carey, J. 1999. "AIDS Drugs: Giving it a Rest." *Business Week.* May 14, 1999 (No. 3633, p. 94).

The Economist. 1999. "A Global Disaster." Jan. 2-8, 1999 (p. 42-44).

The Economist. 1999. "Helping the Poorest." Aug. 14-20, 1999 (p. 11).

The Economist. 2000. "Aid for AIDS." Apr. 29, 2000 (p. 76).

The Economist. 2000. "The Caribbean: Deadly Silence." Apr. 22-28, 2000 (p. 34).

Gellman, B. 2000. "AIDS is Declared Threat to Security." *The Washington Post.* Apr. 30, 2000 (p. A1 and A28).

Gibbings, W. 1999. Rights: "Trinidad and Tobago: Legal Minds Say no to More Laws on AIDS." Inter Press Service (IPS) online (www.ips.org). May 13, 1999.

The Globe and Mail. 1999. "HIV Infection Rate Jumps Sharply in Former USSR." Nov. 24, 1999 (p. A9).

Inter Press Service. 1996. "Jamaica: Health: AIDS Cases Raising Concern." IPS online (www.ips.org). 19 December, 1996.

Inter Press Service. 1997. "Africa: Population: Family Planners Urged to Boost (war against AIDS)." IPS online (www.ips.org). Nov. 24, 1997.

Inter Press Service. 1997. "Trinidad and Tobago: The High Cost of Sex Tourism." IPS online (www.ips.org). 24 March, 1997.

Inter Press Service. 1998. Aegis/Caribbean/37. IPS online (www.ips.org).

Keen, L. 1999. "Is the Goal Control, Through Stop and Go?" *The Washington Blade*. June 4, 1999. Kovaleski, S. 1998. Intolerance, poverty, fuel epidemic of AIDS in Caribbean. *Sunday Start-Times*. Feb. 15, 1998 (p. 15, News).

McNeil Jr., D. 1998. "AIDS Stalking Africa's Struggling Economies." *The New York Times*. Nov. 15, 1998 (p. 1 and 20).

The Miami Herald. 1997. "Dominican Prostitution: Cheap, Prevalent and Accepted." The Miami Herald online (www.miamiherald.com). June 24, 1997.

The Miami Herald. 1998. "Violent Crime Stirs Anxiety in the Caribbean." The Miami Herald online (www.miamiherald.com). Feb. 22, 1998.

The Miami Herald. 1999. "Need for an Effective AIDS Vaccine is Growing More Urgent." The Miami Herald online (www.miamiherald.com). June 11, 1999.

The New York Times. "Gore to Preside at Security Council Session on AIDS Crisis." Jan. 10, 2000 (p. A6).

The New York Times. "Port of Spain Journal: Taking Care of Those who Take Carnival too Far." Mar. 9, 2000 (p. A4).

The Pan African News Agency (PANA). 1999. "Africa: Religious Leaders form Alliance Against AIDS." Integrated Regional Information Network. June 7, 1999.

Reuters Health Information Services. 1999. Lack of education may be barrier to HIV protease inhibitor therapy. May 27, 1999.

Richards, P. 1999. "Rights: Trinidad and Tobago: Children with AIDS Continue to be Shunned." Inter Press Service online (www.ips.org). June 3, 1999.

Russell, S. 1999. "New Crusade to Lower AIDS Drug Costs: Africa's Needs at Odds with Firms' Profit Motive." *San Francisco Chronicle*. May 24, 1999.

Scott, S. 1999. "Some Bars to AIDS Vaccine Lie Outside the Lab." *Baltimore Sun*. May 19, 1999 (p. 1A).

Shillinger, K. 1999. "AIDS and the African." *The Boston Sunday Globe*. Oct. 10, 1999 (p. A1 and A18 and A19).

Stabroek News. 1999. "Religious Leaders Urge Rejection of Violence." Stabroek News online (www.stabroeknews.com). Mar. 10, 1999.

Sykes, R. 2000. "Combining Against the Threat of AIDS." *Financial Times*. Jan. 7, 2000 (p. 17).

The Wall Street Journal. 1999. Volunteers not Hurrying to VaxGen Vaccine Test. June 8, 1999 (p. B13).

The Washington Post. 2000. "AIDS is Declared Threat to Security. White House fears Epidemic Could Destabilize World." April 30, 2000 (p. A1 and A28-29).

The Washington Post. 2000. Cheaper Drugs to Combat AIDS. May 15, 2000 (p. A24).

Distributors of World Bank Group Publications

Prices and credit terms vary from country to country. Consult your local distributor before placing an order.

ARGENTINA
World Publications SA
Av. Cordoba 1877
1120 Ciudad de Buenos Aires
Tel: (54 11) 4815-8156
Fax: (54 11) 4815-8156
E-mail: wpbooks@infovia.com.ar

AUSTRALIA, FIJI, PAPUA NEW GUINEA, SOLOMON ISLANDS, VANUATU, AND SAMOA
D.A. Information Services
648 Whitehorse Road
Mitcham 3132, Victoria
Tel: (61) 3 9210 7777
Fax: (61) 3 9210 7788
E-mail: service@dadirect.com.au
URL: http://www.dadirect.com.au

AUSTRIA
Gerold and Co.
Weihburggasse 26
A-1011 Wien
Tel: (43 1) 512-47-31-0
Fax: (43 1) 512-47-31-29
URL: http://www.gerold.co/at.online

BANGLADESH
Micro Industries Development
Assistance Society (MIDAS)
House 5, Road 16
Dhanmondi R/Area
Dhaka 1209
Tel: (880 2) 326427
Fax: (880 2) 811188

BELGIUM
Jean De Lannoy
Av. du Roi 202
1060 Brussels
Tel: (32 2) 538-5169
Fax: (32 2) 538-0841

BRAZIL
Publicacões Tecnicas Internacionais
Ltda.
Rua Peixoto Gomide, 209
01409 Sao Paulo, SP.
Tel: (55 11) 259-6644
Fax: (55 11) 258-6990
E-mail: postmaster@pti.uol.br
URL: http://www.uol.br

CANADA
Renouf Publishing Co. Ltd.
5369 Canotek Road
Ottawa, Ontario K1J 9J3
Tel: (613) 745-2665
Fax: (613) 745-7660
E-mail:
    order.dept@renoufbooks.com
URL: http:// www.renoufbooks.com

CHINA
China Financial & Economic
    Publishing House
8, Da Fo Si Dong Jie
Beijing
Tel: (86 10) 6401-7365
Fax: (86 10) 6401-7365

China Book Import Centre
P.O. Box 2825
Beijing

Chinese Corporation for Promotion
    of Humanities
52, You Fang Hu Tong,
Xuan Nei Da Jie
Beijing
Tel: (86 10) 660 72 494
Fax: (86 10) 660 72 494

COLOMBIA
Infoenlace Ltda.
Carrera 6 No. 51-21
Apartado Aereo 34270
Santafé de Bogotá, D.C.
Tel: (57 1) 285-2798
Fax: (57 1) 285-2798

COTE D'IVOIRE
Center d'Edition et de Diffusion
    Africaines (CEDA)
04 B.P. 541
Abidjan 04
Tel: (225) 24 6510; 24 6511
Fax: (225) 25 0567

CYPRUS
Center for Applied Research
Cyprus College
6, Diogenes Street, Engomi
P.O. Box 2006
Nicosia
Tel: (357 2) 59-0730
Fax: (357 2) 66-2051

CZECH REPUBLIC
USIS, NIS Prodejna
Havelkova 22
130 00 Prague 3
Tel: (420 2) 2423 1486
Fax: (420 2) 2423 1114
URL: http://www.nis.cz/

DENMARK
SamfundsLitteratur
Rosenoerns Allé 11
DK-1970 Frederiksberg C
Tel: (45 35) 351942
Fax: (45 35) 357822
URL: http://www.sl.cbs.dk

ECUADOR
Libri Mundi
Libreria Internacional
P.O. Box 17-01-3029
Juan Leon Mera 851
Quito
Tel: (593 2) 521-606; (593 2) 544-185
Fax: (593 2) 504-209
E-mail: librimu1@librimundi.com.ec
E-mail: librimu2@librimundi.com.ec

CODEU
Ruiz de Castilla 763, Edif. Expocolor
Primer piso, Of. #2
Quito
Tel/Fax: (593 2) 507-383; 253-091
E-mail: codeu@impsat.net.ec

EGYPT, ARAB REPUBLIC OF
Al Ahram Distribution Agency
Al Galaa Street
Cairo
Tel: (20 2) 578-6083
Fax: (20 2) 578-6833

The Middle East Observer
41, Sherif Street
Cairo
Tel: (20 2) 393-9732
Fax: (20 2) 393-9732

FINLAND
Akateeminen Kirjakauppa
P.O. Box 128
FIN-00101 Helsinki
Tel: (358 0) 121 4418
Fax: (358 0) 121-4435
E-mail: akatilaus@stockmann.fi
URL: http://www.akateeminen.com

FRANCE
Editions Eska; DBJ
48, rue Gay Lussac
75005 Paris
Tel: (33-1) 55-42-73-08
Fax: (33-1) 43-29-91-67

GERMANY
UNO-Verlag
Poppelsdorfer Allee 55
53115 Bonn
Tel: (49 228) 949020
Fax: (49 228) 217492
URL: http://www.uno-verlag.de
E-mail: unoverlag@aol.com

GHANA
Epp Books Services
P.O. Box 44
TUC
Accra
Tel: 223 21 778843
Fax: 223 21 779099

GREECE
Papasotiriou S.A.
35, Stournara Str.
106 82 Athens
Tel: (30 1) 364-1826
Fax: (30 1) 364-8254

HAITI
Culture Diffusion
5, Rue Capois
C.P. 257
Port-au-Prince
Tel: (509) 23 9260
Fax: (509) 23 4858

HONG KONG, CHINA; MACAO
Asia 2000 Ltd.
Sales & Circulation Department
302 Seabird House
22-28 Wyndham Street, Central
Hong Kong, China
Tel: (852) 2530-1409
Fax: (852) 2526-1107
E-mail: sales@asia2000.com.hk
URL: http://www.asia2000.com.hk

HUNGARY
Euro Info Service
Margitszgeti Europa Haz
H-1138 Budapest
Tel: (36 1) 350 80 24, 350 80 25
Fax: (36 1) 350 90 32
E-mail: euroinfo@mail.matav.hu

INDIA
Allied Publishers Ltd.
751 Mount Road
Madras - 600 002
Tel: (91 44) 852-3938
Fax: (91 44) 852-0649

INDONESIA
Pt. Indira Limited
Jalan Borobudur 20
P.O. Box 181
Jakarta 10320
Tel: (62 21) 390-4290
Fax: (62 21) 390-4289

IRAN
Ketab Sara Co. Publishers
Khaled Eslamboli Ave., 6th Street
Delafrooz Alley No. 8
P.O. Box 15745-733
Tehran 15117
Tel: (98 21) 8717819; 8716104
Fax: (98 21) 8712479
E-mail: ketab-sara@neda.net.ir

Kowkab Publishers
P.O. Box 19575-511
Tehran
Tel: (98 21) 258-3723
Fax: (98 21) 258-3723

IRELAND
Government Supplies Agency
Oifig an tSoláthair
4-5 Harcourt Road
Dublin 2
Tel: (353 1) 661-3111
Fax: (353 1) 475-2670

ISRAEL
Yozmot Literature Ltd.
P.O. Box 56055
3 Yohanan Hasandlar Street
Tel Aviv 61560
Tel: (972 3) 5285-397
Fax: (972 3) 5285-397

R.O.Y. International
PO Box 13056
Tel Aviv 61130
Tel: (972 3) 649 9469
Fax: (972 3) 648 6039
E-mail: royil@netvision.net.il
URL: http://www.royint.co.il

Palestinian Authority/Middle East
Index Information Services
P.O.B. 19502 Jerusalem
Tel: (972 2) 6271219
Fax: (972 2) 6271634

ITALY, LIBERIA
Licosa Commissionaria Sansoni SPA
Via Duca Di Calabria, 1/1
Casella Postale 552
50125 Firenze
Tel: (39 55) 645-415
Fax: (39 55) 641-257
E-mail: licosa@ftbcc.it
URL: http://www.ftbcc.it/licosa

JAMAICA
Ian Randle Publishers Ltd.
206 Old Hope Road, Kingston 6
Tel: 876-927-2085
Fax: 876-977-0243
E-mail: irpl@colis.com

JAPAN
Eastern Book Service
3-13 Hongo 3-chome, Bunkyo-ku
Tokyo 113
Tel: (81 3) 3818-0861
Fax: (81 3) 3818-0864
E-mail: orders@svt-ebs.co.jp
URL:
    http://www.bekkoame.or.jp/~svt-ebs

KENYA
Africa Book Service (E.A.) Ltd.
Quaran House, Mfangano Street
P.O. Box 45245
Nairobi
Tel: (254 2) 223 641
Fax: (254 2) 330 272

Legacy Books
Loita House
Mezzanine 1
P.O. Box 68077
Nairobi
Tel: (254) 2-330853, 221426
Fax: (254) 2-330854, 561654
E-mail: Legacy@form-net.com

KOREA, REPUBLIC OF
Dayang Books Trading Co.
International Division
783-20, Pangba Bon-Dong,
Socho-ku
Seoul
Tel: (82 2) 536-9555
Fax: (82 2) 536-0025
E-mail: seamap@chollian.net

Eulyoo Publishing Co., Ltd.
46-1, Susong-Dong
Jongro-Gu
Seoul
Tel: (82 2) 734-3515
Fax: (82 2) 732-9154

LEBANON
Librairie du Liban
P.O. Box 11-9232
Beirut
Tel: (961 9) 217 944
Fax: (961 9) 217 434
E-mail: hsayegh@librairie-du-liban.com.lb
URL: http://www.librairie-du-liban.com.lb

MALAYSIA
University of Malaya Cooperative
    Bookshop, Limited
P.O. Box 1127
Jalan Pantai Baru
59700 Kuala Lumpur
Tel: (60 3) 756-5000
Fax: (60 3) 755-4424
E-mail: umkoop@tm.net.my

MEXICO
INFOTEC
Av. San Fernando No. 37
Col. Toriello Guerra
14050 Mexico, D.F.
Tel: (52 5) 624-2800
Fax: (52 5) 624-2822
E-mail: infotec@rtn.net.mx
URL: http://rtn.net.mx

Mundi-Prensa Mexico S.A. de C.V.
c/Rio Panuco, 141-Colonia
    Cuauhtemoc
06500 Mexico, D.F.
Tel: (52 5) 533-5658
Fax: (52 5) 514-6799

NEPAL
Everest Media International Services
    (P.) Ltd.
GPO Box 5443
Kathmandu
Tel: (977 1) 416 026
Fax: (977 1) 224 431

NETHERLANDS
De Lindeboom/Internationale
    Publicaties b.v.-
P.O. Box 202, 7480 AE Haaksbergen
Tel: (31 53) 574-0004
Fax: (31 53) 572-9296
E-mail: lindeboo@worldonline.nl
URL: http://www.worldonline.nl/~lindeboo

NEW ZEALAND
EBSCO NZ Ltd.
Private Mail Bag 99914
New Market
Auckland
Tel: (64 9) 524-8119
Fax: (64 9) 524-8067

Oasis Official
P.O. Box 3627
Wellington
Tel: (64 4) 499 1551
Fax: (64 4) 499 1972
E-mail: oasis@actrix.gen.nz
URL: http://www.oasisbooks.co.nz/

NIGERIA
University Press Limited
Three Crowns Building Jericho
Private Mail Bag 5095
Ibadan
Tel: (234 22) 41-1356
Fax: (234 22) 41-2056

PAKISTAN
Mirza Book Agency
65, Shahrah-e-Quaid-e-Azam
Lahore 54000
Tel: (92 42) 735 3601
Fax: (92 42) 576 3714

Oxford University Press
5 Bangalore Town
Sharae Faisal
PO Box 13033
Karachi-75350
Tel: (92 21) 446307
Fax: (92 21) 4547640
E-mail: ouppak@TheOffice.net

Pak Book Corporation
Aziz Chambers 21, Queen's Road
Lahore
Tel: (92 42) 636 3222; 636 0885
Fax: (92 42) 636 2328
E-mail: pbc@brain.net.pk

PERU
Editorial Desarrollo SA
Apartado 3824, Ica 242 OF. 106
Lima 1
Tel: (51 14) 285380
Fax: (51 14) 286628

PHILIPPINES
International Booksource Center Inc.
1127-A Antipolo St, Barangay,
    Venezuela
Makati City
Tel: (63 2) 896 6501; 6505; 6507
Fax: (63 2) 896 1741

POLAND
International Publishing Service
Ul. Piekna 31/37
00-677 Warzawa
Tel: (48 2) 628-6089
Fax: (48 2) 621-7255
E-mail: books%ips@ikp.atm.com.pl
URL:
    http://www.ipscg.waw.pl/ips/export

PORTUGAL
Livraria Portugal
Apartado 2681, Rua Do Carm
    o 70-74
1200 Lisbon
Tel: (1) 347-4982
Fax: (1) 347-0264

ROMANIA
Compani De Librarii Bucuresti S.A.
Str. Lipscani no. 26, sector 3
Bucharest
Tel: (40 1) 313 9645
Fax: (40 1) 312 4000

RUSSIAN FEDERATION
Isdatelstvo <Ves Mir>
9a, Kolpachniy Pereulok
Moscow 101831
Tel: (7 095) 917 87 49
Fax: (7 095) 917 92 59
ozimarin@glasnet.ru

**SINGAPORE; TAIWAN, CHINA
MYANMAR; BRUNEI**
Hemisphere Publication Services
41 Kallang Pudding Road #04-03
Golden Wheel Building
Singapore 349316
Tel: (65) 741-5166
Fax: (65) 742-9356
E-mail: ashgate@asianconnect.com

SLOVENIA
Gospodarski vestnik Publishing
    Group
Dunajska cesta 5
1000 Ljubljana
Tel: (386 61) 133 83 47; 132 12 30
Fax: (386 61) 133 80 30
E-mail: repansekj@gvestnik.si

SOUTH AFRICA, BOTSWANA
For single titles:
Oxford University Press Southern
    Africa
Vasco Boulevard, Goodwood
P.O. Box 12119, N1 City 7463
Cape Town
Tel: (27 21) 595 4400
Fax: (27 21) 595 4430
E-mail: oxford@oup.co.za

For subscription orders:
International Subscription Service
P.O. Box 41095
Craighall
Johannesburg 2024
Tel: (27 11) 880-1448
Fax: (27 11) 880-6248
E-mail: iss@is.co.za

SPAIN
Mundi-Prensa Libros, S.A.
Castello 37
28001 Madrid
Tel: (34 91) 4 363700
Fax: (34 91) 5 753998
E-mail: libreria@mundiprensa.es
URL: http://www.mundiprensa.com/

Mundi-Prensa Barcelona
Consell de Cent, 391
08009 Barcelona
Tel: (34 3) 488-3492
Fax: (34 3) 487-7659
E-mail: barcelona@mundiprensa.es

SRI LANKA, THE MALDIVES
Lake House Bookshop
100, Sir Chittampalam Gardiner
    Mawatha
Colombo 2
Tel: (94 1) 32105
Fax: (94 1) 432104
E-mail: LHL@sri.lanka.net

SWEDEN
Wennergren-Williams AB
P. O. Box 1305
S-171 25 Solna
Tel: (46 8) 705-97-50
Fax: (46 8) 27-00-71
E-mail: mail@wwi.se

SWITZERLAND
Librairie Payot Service Institutionnel
C(tm)tes-de-Montbenon 30
1002 Lausanne
Tel: (41 21) 341-3229
Fax: (41 21) 341-3235

ADECO Van Diermen
    EditionsTechniques
Ch. de Lacuez 41
CH1807 Blonay
Tel: (41 21) 943 2673
Fax: (41 21) 943 3605

THAILAND
Central Books Distribution
306 Silom Road
Bangkok 10500
Tel: (66 2) 2336930-9
Fax: (66 2) 237-8321

**TRINIDAD & TOBAGO
AND THE CARRIBBEAN**
Systematics Studies Ltd.
St. Augustine Shopping Center
Eastern Main Road, St. Augustine
Trinidad & Tobago, West Indies
Tel: (868) 645-8466
Fax: (868) 645-8467
E-mail: tobe@trinidad.net

UGANDA
Gustro Ltd.
PO Box 9997, Madhvani Building
Plot 16/4 Jinja Rd.
Kampala
Tel: (256 41) 251 467
Fax: (256 41) 251 468
E-mail: gus@swiftuganda.com

UNITED KINGDOM
Microinfo Ltd.
P.O. Box 3, Omega Park, Alton,
Hampshire GU34 2PG
England
Tel: (44 1420) 86848
Fax: (44 1420) 89889
E-mail: wbank@microinfo.co.uk
URL: http://www.microinfo.co.uk

The Stationery Office
51 Nine Elms Lane
London SW8 5DR
Tel: (44 171) 873-8400
Fax: (44 171) 873-8242
URL: http://www.the-stationery-office.co.uk/

VENEZUELA
Tecni-Ciencia Libros, S.A.
Centro Cuidad Comercial Tamanco
Nivel C2, Caracas
Tel: (58 2) 959 5547; 5035; 0016
Fax: (58 2) 959 5636

ZAMBIA
University Bookshop, University of
    Zambia
Great East Road Campus
P.O. Box 32379
Lusaka
Tel: (260 1) 252 576
Fax: (260 1) 253 952

ZIMBABWE
Academic and Baobab Books (Pvt.)
    Ltd.
4 Conald Road, Graniteside
P.O. Box 567
Harare
Tel: 263 4 755035
Fax: 263 4 781913

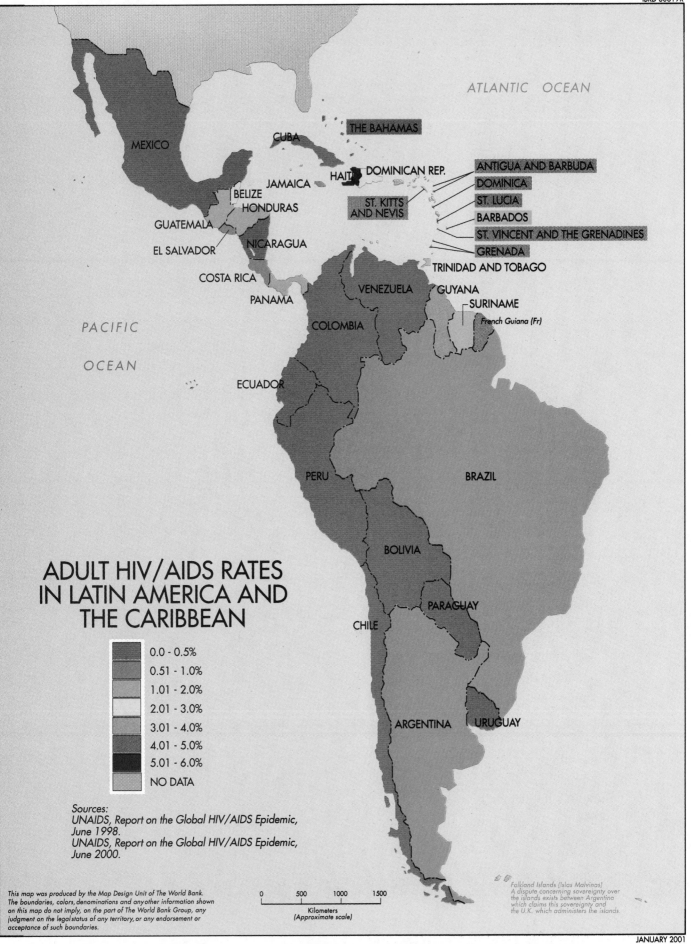

IBRD 30619R

ATLANTIC OCEAN

MEXICO

CUBA

THE BAHAMAS

HAITI   DOMINICAN REP.

ANTIGUA AND BARBUDA

DOMINICA

JAMAICA

BELIZE

HONDURAS

ST. KITTS
AND NEVIS

ST. LUCIA

BARBADOS

GUATEMALA

EL SALVADOR

NICARAGUA

ST. VINCENT AND THE GRENADINES

GRENADA

COSTA RICA

TRINIDAD AND TOBAGO

PANAMA

VENEZUELA

GUYANA

SURINAME

French Guiana (Fr)

PACIFIC

OCEAN

COLOMBIA

ECUADOR

PERU

BRAZIL

BOLIVIA

ADULT HIV/AIDS RATES
IN LATIN AMERICA AND
THE CARIBBEAN

PARAGUAY

CHILE

	0.0 - 0.5%
	0.51 - 1.0%
	1.01 - 2.0%
	2.01 - 3.0%
	3.01 - 4.0%
	4.01 - 5.0%
	5.01 - 6.0%
	NO DATA

ARGENTINA   URUGUAY

Sources:
UNAIDS, Report on the Global HIV/AIDS Epidemic,
June 1998.
UNAIDS, Report on the Global HIV/AIDS Epidemic,
June 2000.

0   500   1000   1500

Kilometers
(Approximate scale)

Falkland Islands (Islas Malvinas)
A dispute concerning sovereignty over
the islands exists between Argentina
which claims this sovereignty and
the U.K. which administers the islands.

JANUARY 2001